WHAT YOU MUST KNOW ABOUT

THYROID
DISORDERS

AND WHAT TO DO ABOUT THEM

WHAT YOU MUST KNOW ABOUT

THYROID
DISORDERS

AND WHAT TO DO ABOUT THEM

SECOND EDITION

PAMELA WARTIAN SMITH, MD, MPH, MS

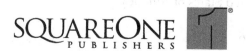

SQUAREONE
PUBLISHERS

EDITOR: Erica Shur
ORIGINAL COVER DESIGN: Jeannie Tudor
TYPESETTING: Gary A. Rosenberg

Square One Publishers
115 Herricks Road
Garden City Park, NY 11040
(516) 535-2010 • (877) 900-BOOK
www.squareonepublishers.com

Library of Congress Cataloging-in-Publication Data
Names: Smith, Pamela Wartian, author.
Title: What you must know about thyroid disorders and what to do about them / Pamela Wartian Smith, MD, MPH, MS.
Description: Second edition. | Garden City Park : Square One Publishers, 2024. | Includes bibliographical references and index.
Identifiers: LCCN 2023031678 | ISBN 9780757005336 (paperback) | ISBN 9780757055331 (ebook)
Subjects: LCSH: Thyroid gland—Diseases—Popular works.
Classification: LCC RC655 .S69 2024 | DDC 616.4/4—dc23/eng/20231023
LC record available at https://lccn.loc.gov/2023031678

Printed in the United States of America

10   9   8   7   6   5   4   3   2

Contents

To Stephen Sinatra, MD.
You were a great mentor in the field of Anti-Aging and Regenerative Medicine. I was so privileged to have been able to be your student, colleague, and friend. Your presence is very much missed by us all.

Acknowledgments

To my publisher Rudy Shur, for his professional direction and commitment, which have helped to make the reading of this book flow smoothly. I am blessed to have the world's best publisher.

To Erica Shur, for continuing to be an amazing editor.

To my husband and best friend, Christopher Smith, whom I am fortunate enough to have as my biggest supporter.

Introduction

All the hormones in the body are a symphony. Much like an orchestra, required to play in tune, your hormonal symphony must be in tune throughout your life in order for you to have optimal health.

Your thyroid gland is more important than you might think. You probably are aware that you have a thyroid gland, but chances are that you may not know the major role it plays in the complex workings of your body. The thyroid gland regulates most everything that occurs in your system. It is, in fact, the conductor of the wonderful symphony that occurs daily in your body. Commonly, it is not until you experience a thyroid dysfunction that you start understanding not only the importance of your thyroid, but also the complexity of how your thyroid affects your well-being. The fact that you are reading this book indicates that you may suspect that you or a loved one has a thyroid problem, or that a specific thyroid issue has already been identified. If that is the case, I believe you've come to the right place. My goal in writing this book is to provide you with an overall understanding of the function of the thyroid gland, the important role the thyroid hormones play in keeping your bodily functions in tune, and the influence the thyroid gland has on your other bodily systems. Just as significant, this book will also offer a closer look at the various problems that arise when the thyroid malfunctions or is not operating optimally.

This book is divided into 18 chapters. Chapter 1 looks at the role the thyroid gland plays as part of the endocrine system—that is, the group of organs and glands responsible for the production of your body's hormones. The text then focuses on the many functions carried on by thyroid hormones and what may occur if they are not at peak levels. Furthermore, just as important is the information contained in this section on how to maintain a healthy thyroid.

In the following chapters we examine specific thyroid disorders. Chapter 2 discusses hypothyroidism, the condition that occurs when the thyroid is underperforming. In Chapter 3, Hashimoto's thyroiditis, which is an autoimmune disease affecting the thyroid, is explored. Chapter 4 examines hyperthyroidism, a condition created when the thyroid produces elevated levels of thyroid hormones. Chapter 5, Graves' disease, the most common form of hyperthyroidism, is reviewed. Likewise, in Chapter 6, provided is information on the lesser-known forms of hyperthyroidism as well as the various disorders caused by, or associated with, hyperthyroidism. Within each of these chapters you will learn about risk factors, causes, and signs and symptoms. You will see how a diagnosis for each disease process is derived, and the treatments used for these thyroid disorders. Whenever possible, a prognosis will be provided, in other words, what the likely outcome will be.

The next chapters deal with the most common and serious health disorders created as a result of thyroid dysfunction. Chapter 7 covers thyroid hormones and your memory; Chapter 8, thyroid hormones and your mood; Chapter 9, thyroid hormones and your heart; Chapter 10, thyroid hormones and hypertension (high blood pressure); and Chapter 11, thyroid hormones and digestive health. In addition, Chapter 12 looks at the thyroid gland and kidney disease; Chapter 13, thyroid and its role in reproductive health; and Chapter 14, thyroid and nonalcoholic fatty liver disease, which is now becoming a common disorder in most industrialized countries including the United States. Moreover, Chapter 15 examines the relationship between thyroid dysfunction and weight gain, Chapter 16 explores thyroid health, diabetes, and insulin resistance, and Chapter 17 reviews COVID-19 and thyroid gland function. As you will discover, the role played by the thyroid hormones interacting with the heart, brain, kidney, liver, digestive system, and other organs is critical to your well being.

In Chapter 18, thyroid cancer is discussed by first explaining what thyroid cancer is. Its risk factors and symptoms are also be elucidated. Because I have found patients can be overwhelmed by not only the situation, but also the medical jargon thrown at them, I will explain the terms commonly used to describe the test, characteristics of the cells, the stages, and the treatments provided. I will then discuss each of the most common thyroid cancers. For every single one, I will include risk factors, causes, and signs and symptoms. In addition, I will describe how each is diagnosed, its standard treatments, and its prognosis.

By the end of this book, as you will come to see, although relatively small, the thyroid gland plays many vital roles in the human body. Through its release of hormones, it helps regulate heart rate, breathing, digestion, body temperature, weight, mood, memory, and so much more. It is my hope that the information in this book will provide you with all the important facts you may be looking for you to achieve and maintain optimal health.

1

You and Your Thyroid

How important is your thyroid gland to your overall health, and what could go wrong with your thyroid gland? What hormones does your thyroid gland produce, and why are they so important? This chapter will address these questions and help you understand how your thyroid gland regulates almost all functions that occur in your body through the production of several hormones. You'll learn how it is instrumental in regulating the body's metabolism and calcium usage; and how it affects your brain development, muscle control, heart, and digestive function, as well as bone maintenance. The thyroid gland can become overactive (hyperthyroidism) or underactive (hypothyroidism), which affects your well-being, resulting in several issues, such as weight gain or loss, fatigue, intolerance of hot or cold temperatures, and depression or anxiety.

You will discover how this butterfly-shaped gland regulates almost everything that occurs in your body. A healthy thyroid is essential in order for you to have optimal health. By understanding how the thyroid functions and the various components of the thyroid gland, you will gain insight into the problems created when the thyroid isn't working optimally.

The thyroid affects many organ systems in the body. Thyroid hormone induces effects on practically all nucleated cells in the human body, generally increasing their function and metabolism.

THE ENDOCRINE SYSTEM

The endocrine system is composed of glands and organs (see Figure 1.1 on page 6), which produce important chemical agents called hormones. This includes the adrenal glands, ovaries, pancreas, parathyroid, pineal gland, pituitary gland, hypothalamus, ovaries and testes, thymus, and thyroid gland, as well as the stomach, small intestines, liver, kidneys, and skin.

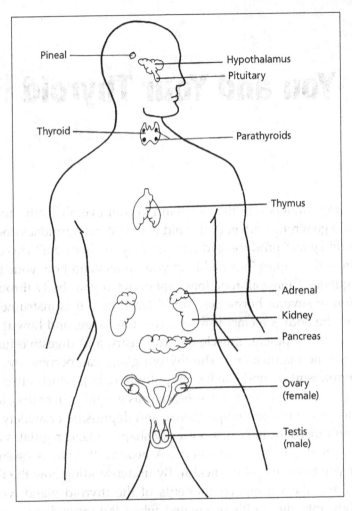

Figure 1.1. The Endocrine System

The hormones produced by the endocrine system regulate the activities of cells and organs in order to help your body function properly. This is done by releasing the hormones directly into the blood stream. When any of these glands or organs lose their ability to produce hormones properly, this can lead to thyroid disease, diabetes, growth disorders, sexual dysfunction, and other serious health issues.

The hormones released into the blood stream by the glands of the endocrine system are specific to each gland. Each gland performs by releasing hormones that aid in coordinating the body processes.

- Adrenal glands release cortisol and DHEA.

- Hypothalamus produces gonadotropin-releasing hormone (GnRH) and prompts the pituitary gland to release hormones (prolactin, follicle-stimulating hormone (FSH), luteinizing hormone (LH)). It also produces oxytocin, which plays a role in social bonding, reproduction, childbirth, and milk production.

- Ovaries release eggs and produce the sex hormones (estrogen, progesterone, and testosterone).

- Pancreas releases the hormones from both the endocrine and exocrine systems.

- The endocrine pancreas hormones include the following:

  o **VIP, or Vasoactive Intestinal Peptide Hormone:** It aids you in the control of water absorption and secretion from the intestines by stimulating the islets of Langerhans to release salt and water into the intestine.

  o **Glucagon:** It helps in maintaining normal blood sugar by working in tandem with the insulin, although in a different direction.

  o **Gastrin Hormone:** It helps in digestion as well as stimulating various cells in the stomach in order to produce acid that aids in digestion.

  o **Somatostatin Hormone:** It is of use whenever the levels of other pancreatic hormones, such as glucagon or insulin, become elevated. This hormone is indeed secreted in order to maintain a balance of salt and sugar in the blood.

  o **Insulin** secreted by the pancreas aids in regulating blood sugar by allowing many of the blood cells to absorb and use blood sugar, hence dropping the blood sugar levels.

- The exocrine pancreas hormones include:

  o **Cholecystokinin** is a hormone that is secreted by cells in the duodenum and stimulates the release of bile into the intestine and the secretion of enzymes by the pancreas.

- Parathyroid is crucial to bone development and releases parathyroid hormone, which helps to control the levels of calcium, phosphorus, and magnesium in the body.

- Pineal gland is linked to patterns of sleep, since it releases the hormone melatonin.

- Pituitary gland influences many glands, most importantly the thyroid, ovaries, and testes. It produces the hormones FSH, LH, prolactin, TSH (thyroid stimulating hormone), ACTH (a hormone that stimulates the adrenal glands), and growth hormone.

- Testes produce sperm and sex hormones such as testosterone made in the Leydig cells. The testes also make these other hormones.

  o **Inhibin B**: Serum levels of this protein are related to testicular volume and sperm counts in adults.

  o **Anti-Mullerian hormone**: This hormone is important to the development of internal male reproductive organs.

  o **Insulin-like Hormone 3 (INSL3):** This hormone helps testicles descend into the scrotum from the abdomen and to continue to develop in the scrotum.

  o **Estradiol**: This hormone is important in making sperm as well as cognitive function and helping to maintain bone structure.

- Thymus helps in the development of the immune system early on in life.

- Thyroid controls many aspects of your metabolism, as you will learn.

FUNCTIONS OF THE THYROID GLAND AND THYROID HORMONES IN YOUR BODY

The thyroid gland is a key gland, producing hormones that play a major part in the human body's everyday workings. These hormones:

- Affect tissue repair and development

- Aid in the function of the mitochondria (energy makers of your cells)

- Assist in the digestion process by regulating GI tone and motility

- Control hormone secretion and therefore regulates fertility, ovulation, and menstruation

- Control oxygen utilization by regulating resting respiratory rate and minute ventilation

- Modulate blood flow

- Regulate carbohydrate, protein, and lipid metabolism

- Modulate muscle and nerve action

- Modulate sexual function

- Regulate energy and heat production through blood flow, sweating, and ventilation

- Regulate growth and repair

- Regulate vitamin usage, for example, by promoting folate (B9) and cobalamin (B12) absorption through the GI tract

- Regulate cardiac output, stroke volume, contractility, and resting heart rate

- Regulate metabolic rate (BMR)

- Promote oxygen delivery to the tissues by simulating erythropoietin and hemoglobin production

- Stimulate the nervous system, resulting in increased wakefulness, alertness, and responsiveness to external stimuli

- Stimulate the peripheral nervous system, resulting in increased peripheral reflexes

- Responsible for the development of fetal growth centers and liner bone growth

- Renal (kidney) clearance of many substances, including medications can be increased due to an increase in renal blood flow and glomerular filtration rate

- Increase development of type II muscle fibers

Description

Your thyroid gland is one of the largest endocrine glands. It is a ductless gland, butterfly in shape, consisting of two connected lobes (two wings), attached by the isthmus, located in the front of the neck below your Adam's apple, and it is wrapped around the trachea (the windpipe). It is the biggest gland in your neck. It has a brownish-red color as a result of the rich blood vessels located in the thyroid gland. When normal in size, you can't feel it. The thyroid is what sets the speed at, which your body operates. It reminds your cells to function at a certain rate.

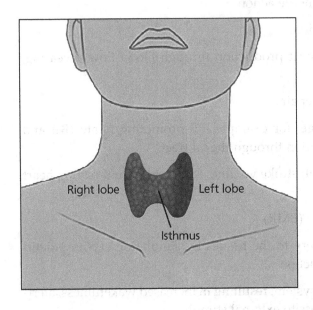

Figure 1.2.
The Thyroid Gland

Right lobe

Left lobe

Isthmus

Source: National Cancer Institute

The Thyroid Cells

A healthy thyroid is composed of several specialized cells. Many of these cells produce a number of hormones, which perform different tasks. Each thyroid cell capable of producing a specific hormone has within it different structures that can identify what type of cell it is, as seen in Table 1.1.

TABLE 1.1. THE NORMAL THYROID CELLS AND THEIR FUNCTION	
Thyroid Cells	**Function**
Follicular cells and (epithelial or principal cells)	Cells in the thyroid gland that have control over the production discharge of thyroid hormones thyroxine (T4) and triiodothyronine (T3). These cells are found lining the surface of the thyroid.
Parafollicular Cells (C cells)	Cells that secrete calcitonin (a hormone that regulates calcium metabolism), located in the spaces between the spherical follicles. These cells are large, located in the connective tissue of the thyroid.
Endothelial cells	Cells that are found in the lining of the blood vessels that run through the thyroid.

Hormones and Their Functions

Hormones are chemical agents manufactured by the body. They are produced by specific glands and are secreted into the blood, and then transported by the circulatory system to the areas of the body where they impact cells and organs. Having normal thyroid function relies heavily on the thyroid hormones T2 (3,5-Diiodo-L-thyronine), T3 (Triiodothyronine), T4 (Thyroxine), and rT3 (reverse triiodothyronine) secreted by the thyroid gland. The pituitary gland, located in the brain, is instrumental in the production of these hormones by providing a signal in the form of thyroid stimulating hormone (TSH).

The process begins when the hypothalamus gland, located in the brain, produces the hormone thyrotrophin-releasing hormone (TRH). This, in turn, stimulates the pituitary gland, also located in the brain, to produce TSH. From the pituitary gland, the TSH travels to the thyroid in order to regulate the production and control the release of each of the thyroid hormones that the body produces. There are several different thyroid hormones that your body synthesizes. They are:

- Diiodothyronine (T2)
- Triiodothyronine (T3)
- Thyroxine (T4)
- Reverse triiodothyronine (rT3)

T2. T2 increases the metabolic rate of your muscles and fat tissues. T2 stimulates cellular/mitochondrial respiration and outside the cell affects the carriers, ion-exchanges, and enzymes. It may also affect the transcription of genes.

T3. This hormone is four to five times more active than T4. T3 is about 20 percent of the thyroid hormone production by the body. It affects most of the physiological processes in the body except for those in the spleen and testes. This hormone increases basal metabolic rate, oxygen, and energy consumption by the body. It is very important for weight loss and to breakdown cholesterol. It even affects the production of serotonin in the brain, which is your happy neurotransmitter. T3 furthermore increases the rate of protein synthesis and affects glucose metabolism. The T3 hormone is available in two forms: bound T3, which is attached to protein, and free T3, which does not attach to anything. When you have your T3 measured, your healthcare provider should measure the free form.

T4. T4 is 80 percent of the thyroid gland's production. Most of T4 is converted into T3 in your liver or kidneys, so some authors suggest that T4

Conversion of T4 to T3

The hormones T3 and T4 are produced by the follicular cells. The hormone T4 is in "storage" in your body, and in order for your body to use T4 it must first change it to the active hormone T3. Deficiencies of zinc, copper, vitamins A, B_2, B_3, B_6, and C are factors that cause decreased production of T4, which leads to symptoms of hypothyroidism. Consequently, in order for thyroid function to be optimal, your body must easily convert T4 to the more active T3. The conversion of T4 to T3 requires the enzyme 5'deiodinase, which plays a role in the activation or deactivation of thyroid hormones. There are three types of 5'deiodinases enzymes, which can deiodinate (remove iodine) thyroid hormones.

- Type I (D1), which is located in the thyroid, liver, and kidney is involved in the production of T3 by converting inactive T4 to active T3. It has been found to have reduced activity in patients with hypothyroidism.

- Type II (D2), which is found in the pituitary, hypothalamus, and brown fat converts T4 to T3. It is also expressed in skeletal muscle, heart, and thyroid. It produces the majority of circulating T3. D2 is also found to be increased in hypothyroid and iodine-deficient individuals.

- Type III (D3), which catalyzes deiodination of the inner ring of T4 to T3 and inactivates the hormone (reverse T3). It is found primarily in the placenta, skin, skeletal muscle, and the developing brain. It is essential for sensory development, particularly within the inner ear.

As mentioned above deiodinase enzymes are important in the activation or deactivation of thyroid hormones. The following elements negatively affect the production of 5'deiodinase:

- Cadmium, mercury, and lead toxicity
- Chronic illness
- Decreased kidney or liver function
- Elevated cortisol
- High carbohydrate diet
- Inadequate protein intake
- Inflammation
- Selenium deficiency
- Starvation
- Stress

There are numerous factors that affect the conversion of T4 to the more active T3. Although many physicians may prescribe T4 to manage the condition, often this isn't enough. To correct the conversion problem, you need to determine what is causing the issue. The following are some common factors that can impede the conversion of T4 to T3.

Nutritional deficiencies

Certain minerals and nutrients are needed to activate enzymes, such as iron, iodine, selenium, zinc, vitamins A, B_2, B_6, and B_{12}.

Medications

Some medications can interfere with the conversion of T4 to T3. For example:

- Beta blockers
- Clomipramine
- Estrogen replacement
- Glucocorticoids
- Interleukin (IL-6)
- Lithium
- Oral contraceptives
- Some chemotherapeutic agents
- Theophylline

Diet

Your diet may be a crucial element in the conversion process as well and can negatively impact thyroid production.

- Eating too many walnuts
- Excessive alcohol use
- Low carbohydrate diet
- Low fat diet
- Low protein diet
- Large amount of soy
- Too many cruciferous vegetables (broccoli, cauliflower, kale, Brussels sprouts)

Other factors that inhibit the T4 to T3 conversion

- Aging process
- Calcium excess
- Copper excess
- Diabetes
- Dioxins
- Fluoride
- High dose alpha lipoic acid (600 mg and above)
- Inadequate production of DHEA and/or cortisol
- Lead
- Mercury
- PCBs
- Pesticides
- Phthalates (chemicals added to plastics)
- Radiation
- Stress
- Surgery

is really a prohormone (a steroid). T4 is responsible for increasing cardiac output, increasing basal metabolic rate, and increasing heart rate and ventilation. It also potentiates the effect of catecholamines (type of hormone that strongly affects blood pressure) and thickens the endometrium of the uterus in women. T4 can also be converted into rT3, which is an inactive (stored) form. The T4 hormone is also available in two forms: bound T4, which is attached to protein, and free T4, which is not bound. When you have your T4 measured, your healthcare provider should measure the free form.

rT3. Reverse T3 is produced from T4, and its function is to block the action of T3. Furthermore, it affects the body's ability to store T3 for use at another time. High reverse T3 slows down the metabolism by attaching to the cell receptor sites for the free T3. Therefore, free T3 cannot get into the cell and optimize its function. Reverse T3 acts like a key in the keyhole (receptors) of the cell. It is impossible to put a free T3 key into a keyhole that already has a different key in it (reverse T3). In other words, with the wrong key, the engine of the car will not start, and the cell will not get the required free T3 to function properly. Consequently, reverse T3 is a break on thyroid function and metabolism. Stored reverse T3 means you cannot use it and even though your level of free T3 may be within the normal range, you still may experience symptoms of hypothyroidism (low thyroid function).

Chronic stress (as well as the factors that follow) causes the adrenal glands to manufacture a high level of cortisol, which hinders the conversion of T4 to T3 and may result in an increased level of rT3 since it is a measurement of inactive thyroid function. Your rT3 has only 1 percent of the activity T3 does. It is an antagonist of T3, which means that the higher your rT3 level is, the lower your T3 level will be. As previously discussed, T3 and rT3 bind to the same receptor sites, so they cannot both occupy these sites at the same time. This situation occurs due to a malfunction of the metabolism of T4. The following are factors that are associated with low T3 or increased reverse T3:

- Aggressive exercise programs without replenishment of nutrients

- Aging process

- Diabetes

- Elevated levels of IL-6, TNF alpha, IFN-2

- Fasting or dieting

- Free radical production

- Hidden gut infections/parasites
- Increased levels of epinephrine and/or norepinephrine
- Inflammation
- Long-haul COVID
- Low iron (ferritin) levels
- Prolonged illness
- Stress
- Toxic metal exposure

When rT3 is high, it results in a medical syndrome now called "rT3 dominance."

Causes of rT3 Dominance

rT3 dominance, also known as Wilson's Syndrome, is a condition that exhibits hypothyroid symptoms although circulating levels of T3 and T4 are within normal test limits. Some of the causes of this condition include:

- Autoimmune disease
- Exposure to electromagnetic radiation
- Exposure to environmental toxins, such as chemical pollutants, pesticides, mercury, or fluoride
- Food deprivation
- High levels of stress
- Hormonal imbalance (such as high estrogen levels in women)
- Infections
- Nutritional deficiencies
- Poor liver function

Furthermore, high normal or elevated rT3 is indicative of reduced thyroid transport. It may cause your metabolism to slow down, affecting your body temperature, fatigue, and eating habits. This may be due to mitochondrial dysfunction. Your body needs energy to carry out its many jobs. Mitochondria are literally an energy factory. The mitochondria produce 90 percent of the energy your body needs to function. The job of the mitochondria is to process oxygen and convert substances from the food you eat into energy. Mitochondria occur in nearly all cells in the body. If you suffer from mitochondrial dysfunction, then the mitochondria are not changing nutrients into energy, and therefore needed energy is not produced.

Hence, any disease process associated with mitochondrial dysfunction may be associated with high normal or elevated rT3. There are several conditions that have been found to be commonly associated with elevated rT3.

- Aging
- Anxiety
- Bipolar depression
- Cardiovascular disease
- Chronic and acute dieting
- Chronic fatigue syndrome
- Chronic infections
- Depression
- Diabetes
- Fibromyalgia

- Hypercholesterolemia (high cholesterol) and hypertriglyceridemia (high triglycerides)
- Inflammation and chronic illnesses
- Insulin resistance
- Long-haul COVID
- Migraines
- Neurodegenerative disorders such as Parkinson's disease and Alzheimer's disease
- Obesity

In addition, rT3 has been shown to have a direct effect on the proliferation of human glioblastoma and breast cancer cell lines. It increases proliferation in vitro of 50 percent to 80 percent of these cells. Therefore, rT3 may be a host factor supporting cancer growth.

The transporter for T4 is more energy dependent than the transporter for T3. Cellular levels of thyroid are not detected well by serum T4 levels, since serum T4 is transported into the cell and the lower the cellular level of T4 the higher the serum level. The most important determinant of thyroid activity is the intra-cellular T3 level. High normal or elevated rT3 levels are the best measure of suboptimal thyroid transport into the cell. Furthermore, consider looking at free T3 to rT3 ratio. The optimal ratio of freeT3 to reverse T3 should be greater than 20. If your ratio is 20 or less, then too much of your free T3 is converting into rT3.

How To Lower Reverse T3

Excess rT3 (stored thyroid hormone) will further inhibit conversion from T4 to T3. Free T3 and rT3 occupy the same receptor sites. However, T3 will activate the receptor, rT3 will not. If rT3 is high, you may have symptoms of hypothyroidism, even if your labs are normal. There are several ways to lower elevated reverse T3 levels.

- Since rT3 is derived from T4, your doctor can lower the T4 dose or discontinue the T4

- Your doctor can prescribe T3. T3 will lower the TSH and subsequent production of T4 by the thyroid gland and inappropriate conversion to rT3

- Eliminate stress

- Treat selenium deficiency

- Treat iodine deficiency

- Treat infection if present

- Treat underlying mitochondrial problem by supplementing with these nutrients:

  ○ Magnesium

  ○ Coenzyme Q-10

  ○ Alpha lipoic acid

  ○ L-carnitine (if your TMAO level is normal)

  ○ NADH (NAD + hydrogen) or NAD+ (nicotinamide adenine dinucleotide)

  ○ D-ribose

- Growth hormone replacement (last resort)

Lab Studies to Evaluate Thyroid Function

Conditions that interfere with the normal process of the thyroid gland are categorized as influencing the thyroid directly or indirectly. Blood tests are readily available and widely used to measure thyroid function and identify the most common causes of thyroid dysfunction. Blood analyses are used to determine whether your thyroid is functioning properly. It is very important that you have optimal levels of thyroid hormone and not just normal levels. See Table 1.2 on page 18 for a list of your normal thyroid hormones based on your blood test, as well as the optimal range of thyroid hormone for each lab.

TABLE 1.2. THYROID FUNCTION TEST INTERPRETATION		
Test	Optimal Range*	Possible Diagnosis
TSH	0.35 mU/L to 2.0 mU/L	High TSH indicates an underactive thyroid (hypothyroidism)
		Low TSH indicates an overactive thryroid (hyperthyroidism)
Free T4	0.8 ng/dL to 1.8 ng/dL	Levels are low (hypothyroidism)
		Levels are elevated (hyperthyroidism)
Free T3	2.0 pg/mL to 4.2 pg/mL	Levels are elevated (hyperthyroidism)
		Levels are low (hypothyroidism)
rT3	10 ng/dL to 22 ng/dL	High normal (22 to 24 ng/dL) or elevated (triggered by chronic stress, pneumonia, injury, surgery, low iron, or low cortisol) (hypothyroidism or hyperthyroidism)
Thyroid antibodies		Normal range should be negative
Antithyroglobulin	Negative	Positive indicates Hashimoto's thyroiditis
Antimicrosomal	Negative	Positive indicates Hashimoto's thyroiditis, autoimmune hemolytic anemia, Graves' disease, Sjögren syndrome, systemic lupus erythematosus, rheumatoid arthritis, and/or thyroid cancer
Antithyroperoxidase (ATPO)	Negative	Positive indicates Hashimoto's thyroiditis, Graves' disease, Sjögren's syndrome, lupus, rheumatoid arthritis, and/or pernicious anemia
Thyroid-stimulating Hormone (TSH) receptor	Negative	Positive indicates Graves' disease

*Normal range may vary from lab to lab.

Standard Blood Test. Normally, every blood test you take includes a group of tests that look at your body's hormones. It typically analyzes your thyroid hormones, including TSH, free T3, free T4, reverse T3; thyroid antibodies; antithyroglobulin; antimicrosomal; antithyroperoxidase; and the thyroid-stimulating hormone receptor. The results are printed on your blood test lab report.

- Thyroid-stimulating hormone (TSH). It measures the amount of TSH in the blood. TSH is produced by the pituitary gland and is located in the brain. It is responsible for regulating the amount of hormones released by the thyroid gland.

- Free T3 and Free T4. These levels measure the free hormone in the blood, which is not bound and able to enter and affect the body tissues.

- Reverse T3. This level is the body's ability to store free T3 for a "rainy day." Stored Reverse T3 means you cannot use it and even though your level of free T3 could be within the normal range, you still may experience hypothyroid symptoms.

- Thyroid antibodies.

Thyroid Binding Globulin Test (TBG). TBG is a protein that's produced by the liver. Its purpose is to bind to thyroid hormones, T4 and T3. and carry them through your bloodstream. This test is specifically administered to find the reason for elevated or diminished levels of thyroid hormone. TBG levels don't mean much in cases of hypothyroidism or hyperthyroidism due to actual dysfunction of the thyroid gland. They do, however, become especially important if you have abnormal levels of T3 or T4 but no symptoms of thyroid dysfunction.

If the TBG level is high, for example, the TBG binds to more thyroid hormone, and that leaves less of the free hormone circulating in the blood. That leads the body to put out more thyroid-stimulating hormone, which leads to the production of more thyroid hormone. Therefore, the total thyroid hormone level will be elevated even though you do not have hyperthyroidism.

Elevated TBG levels may be caused by the following:

- Hypothyroidism
- Liver disease
- Acute intermittent porphyria
- Genetics
- Pregnancy
- Estrogen replacement therapy
- Oral contraceptives
- Other medications

Low TBG levels may be caused by:

- Hyperthyroidism
- Kidney disease
- Liver disease
- Acromegaly (abnormal growth of the hands, feet, and face)

- Malnutrition
- Certain medications
- Cushing's syndrome
- Severe illness

Thyrotropin-releasing Hormone Test (TRH). This test is specifically to find the levels of the thyrotropin-releasing hormone, also called thyrotropin releasing factor (TRF), which is produced by the hypothalamus. TRF:

- Stimulates the release of TSH and prolactin from the pituitary

- Is the central regulator of the hypothalamic-pituitary-thyroid (HPT) axis

- Has affects independent of the HPT axis

- Protects the neurons against oxidative stress, glutamate toxicity, caspase-induced cell death, DNA fragmentation, and inflammation

- Is involved in immune regulation

In addition, as you age, the body commonly produces less TRH, which is implicated in neurodegenerative diseases (Alzheimer's and Parkinson's).

Total T4 and Total T3. These levels measure bound and free thyroid hormones in the blood. The levels are influenced by many things that affect protein levels in the body, such as medications, sex hormones, and liver disease. For optimal health, your total T3 to reverse T3 ratio should be greater than 10.

MAINTAINING A HEALTHY THYROID GLAND

Although many thyroid disorders may be genetic, you can greatly *reduce* the risk of developing any thyroid malfunctions by paying close attention to the foods you eat, making sure you get enough exercise, and avoiding as many toxins as you can.

Diet

A diet that is balanced and rich in vitamin A, iodine, selenium, and iron will aid in hormone production. To increase your selenium intake, choose foods such as Brazil nuts, shellfish, mushrooms, wheat germ, sunflower and sesame seeds, onion, garlic, beef liver, and eggs. The daily recommended dose of these important nutrients is as follows:

- Vitamin A: 4,000 IU daily

- Iodine: Individuals age 14 and older, 15 mcg daily

- Iron: For men, 8 mg daily; for women, 18 mg up to menopause, after menopause take 8 mg daily

- Selenium: Daily dose 55 mcg, however try to get the daily requirement from the foods listed above

Considerations

- Sugar intake interferes with a balanced diet, since sugar provides "empty calories." Sugar can reduce thyroid function, lower circulation, and also cause weight gain.

- Polyunsaturated oils should be limited as well, as they affect hormone and progesterone production. Replacing polyunsaturated oils with coconut oil is a healthy choice.

- Monitor foods that suppress the function of the thyroid gland by interfering with the absorption of iodine, for example green cruciferous vegetables (broccoli, Brussels sprouts, collard greens, spinach, kale, and others), as well as certain fruits, such as peaches, pears, and strawberries. These foods should be eaten in moderation unless you already have a low iodine level.

Exercise

Physical activity is instrumental in achieving a healthy body weight, it will decrease stress levels, increase lean muscle mass, and provide you with more energy. Aerobic exercise can raise your levels of T3 and T4, for those who suffer from low levels of thyroid hormones, and boost your metabolism. A regular exercise program and staying active is important for circulation, which is essential in assisting the thyroid in the distribution of hormones.

Limiting Exposure to Synthetic Hormones

Many people do not realize that they encounter synthetic hormones and hormone-like chemicals in daily living. For example, synthetic estrogen may be derived from animal estrogen. The body recognizes these type of hormones as foreign substances and does not metabolize them well.

Unfortunately, there are a number of synthetic hormones in the things that you come into contact with every day that may have a detrimental effect on your thyroid health. Xenoestrogens are a type of synthetic hormone that imitates estrogen and has been implicated in many conditions. They pass into the environment and into your body through certain foods, plastics, certain chemicals, and household and personal products.

Synthetic hormones may increase your risk of developing heart disease, breast cancer, ovarian cancer, high blood pressure, and so on. You cannot totally avoid xenoestrogens, but you can lessen their effect and the chances of being exposed to them.

Considerations

- Drinking filtered water rather than tap water
- Eating organic foods that have not been exposed to pesticides and herbicides rather than processed foods that may contain preservatives and synthetic hormones
- Using natural detergents and body care products
- Decreasing caffeine intake may improve your thyroid function
- Using organic household cleaning products

Annual Medical Check-Ups

Diet, exercise, and limiting exposure to synthetic hormones can help you maintain a healthy thyroid and alleviate the symptoms of some thyroid conditions, but it should not be a substitute for a medical examination and blood test. By learning what the signs and symptoms of the most common thyroid problems are, you will be in a better position to have them evaluated by your physician and catch it early enough to stop it from causing serious harm to your body. In Table 1.3 on page 23 you will find the most common thyroid disorders that are often related to an over- or an under-functioning thyroid.

Hypothyroidism and hyperthyroidism can then be divided into subsets: overt and subclinical hypothyroidism and overt and subclinical hyperthyroidism. Subclinical hypothyroidism happens when you have elevated thyroid-stimulating hormone (TSH) levels with normal thyroxine levels. Subclinical hyperthyroidism is defined by a low or undetectable serum thyroid-stimulating hormone level, with normal free thyroxine and free triiodothyronine levels. The following diagram depicts these different classes of abnormal thyroid function, which will be discussed in subsequent chapters of this book.

TABLE 1.3. DISORDERS AND THEIR RELATED HORMONE ISSUES	
Disorder	Hormone Issue
Goiter	Iodine deficiency, excess production of thyroid hormone, Hashimoto's Thyroiditis Low production of thyroid hormone
Hyperthyroidism	High production of thyroid hormone
Hypothyroidism	Low production of thyroid hormone
Graves' Disease	Excess production of thyroid hormone
Thyroid Cancer	Iodine deficiency, low level of thyroid hormone promotes higher production of TSH, which promotes growth of thyroid cancer cells (See Chapter 18.)
Thyroid Nodule	Excess of thyroid hormone, diets deficient in iodine
Thyroid Storm	Excess of thyroid hormone, over-replacement of thyroid emergency hormone

CONCLUSION

As you can see, your thyroid gland is one of the most important glands in your body since it is the conductor of your body's symphony. To achieve optimal health, your thyroid gland, along with your hypothalamus and pituitary gland, which help regulate thyroid hormone production, must all be functioning perfectly. In the next chapter you will learn about the causes, symptoms, and the treatment of a low-functioning thyroid gland, a condition referred to as hypothyroidism.

2

Hypothyroidism

Hypothyroidism—an underactive thyroid—is a more common disorder than you may think. As of 2021, in the United States, 1 in 300 people have been diagnosed with hypothyroidism. Of these, around 80 percent of them are women. People of any age can suffer from hypothyroidism, but it is more common in older adults. It is seven times more common in females than in males, and women over the age of 50 are at a higher risk. While hypothyroidism can take several forms, the most common is Hashimoto's thyroiditis. (See page 55 for details.)

CONDITIONS ASSOCIATED WITH HYPOTHYROIDISM

- Iodine deficiency

- Cretinism (severe deficiency of thyroid hormone in newborns)

- Wolff-Chaikoff effect (presumed reduction in thyroid hormone levels caused by ingestion of a large amount of iodine)

- Subacute thyroiditis

- Postpartum thyroiditis (thyroid gland becomes inflamed after having a baby)

- Riedel thyroiditis (rare chronic inflammatory disease of the thyroid characterized by a dense fibrosis that replaces normal thyroid parenchyma)

- Hashimoto's thyroiditis

- Drug-induced

As previously noted, clinical hypothyroidism affects 1 in 300 people in the Unites States with women more commonly affected than men.

Hypothyroidism is defined as low thyroid function or an underactive thyroid, where the thyroid gland does not make enough thyroid hormones to allow the body to function optimally. The main function of the thyroid hormone is to oversee your metabolism, therefore people with this condition have symptoms associated with a low-functioning metabolism. Hypothyroidism disturbs the normal equilibrium of the chemical reactions in the body. Unfortunately, the earliest signs and symptoms of low thyroid function can occur several years prior to laboratory results being abnormal. It is therefore important to be aware of this disorder's signs and symptoms.

Overt or clinical primary hypothyroidism is defined as thyroid-stimulating hormone (TSH) concentrations above the reference range and free T4 and/or free T3 concentrations below the reference range. Mild or subclinical hypothyroidism, which is commonly regarded as a sign of early hypothyroidism, is defined by TSH concentrations above the reference range and free T4 and/or free T3 concentrations within the normal range.

RISK FACTORS

There are several risk factors that can increase the possibility of developing hypothyroidism. The following elements may indicate if an individual is at increased risk.

Age

Although hypothyroidism can occur at any age, women over the age of 60 are more likely to develop hypothyroidism.

Autoimmune Disorders

Medical research has found that 90 percent of people produce antibodies that attack and destroy thyroid tissue. This process over time limits the amount of thyroid hormones being produced, which leads to hypothyroidism.

Ethnicity

Statistically, whites and Asians appear to be at greater risk for hypothyroidism than other people.

Genetics

Statistics strongly indicate that genetics plays a role in a person's predisposition to developing hypothyroidism. While there is no evidence that only one gene is to blame, it is more likely that the presence of several specific genes increases the incidence of hypothyroidism. However, in order to turn these genes on, it may require one or more triggers, as listed below, to initiate this condition.

Gender

Women are at a higher risk of developing hypothyroidism then men.

Smoking

Smoking has been found to be associated with lower levels of total T4 in females.

CAUSES

There are two forms of hypothyroidism: primary hypothyroidism, which is due to a problem with the thyroid gland itself and central or secondary hypothyroidism, which may be congenital (present at birth) or acquired in childhood or adulthood due to hypothalamic or pituitary disease or injury.

Central hypothyroidism is rare and occurs when there is insufficient production of bioactive TSH due to pituitary or hypothalamic tumors (including craniopharyngiomas), infiltrative, inflammatory (lymphocytic or granulomatous hypophysitis), hemorrhagic necrosis (Sheehan's syndrome), or iatrogenic (illness causes by medical examination or treatment) disorders of the pituitary or hypothalamus. Genetic disorders with distinct genetic syndromes with multiple autoimmune endocrinopathies have been described, with some overlapping clinical features. The presence of two of the three major characteristics is required to diagnose the syndrome of multiple autoimmune endocrinopathies (MAEs). The defining major characteristics for type 1 MAE and type 2 MAE are as follows:

- Type 1 MAE: Hypoparathyroidism, Addison's disease, and mucocutaneous candidiasis caused by mutations in the autoimmune regulator gene (AIRE), resulting in defective AIRE protein. Autoimmune thyroiditis is present in about 1 percent to 15 percent.

- Type 2 MAE: Addison's disease, autoimmune thyroiditis, and type 1 diabetes known as Schmidt's syndrome.

An estimated 1 in 13,000 people have central hypothyroidism. About 60 percent are part of combined pituitary hormone deficiencies.

Primary hypothyroidism is the more common form of hypothyroidism and may be due to a number of other factors, such as diet, Hashimoto's thyroiditis (see page 55), an unhealthy gut, thyroid surgery (partial or total thyroidectomy), radiation therapy, and medications (e.g., amiodarone and lithium), as well as deficiencies in certain minerals and vitamins, which are factors that cause decreased production of T4 and lead to symptoms of hypothyroidism. Other causes include transient hypothyroidism due to silent thyroiditis, subacute thyroiditis, or postpartum thyroiditis. The remainder of this chapter will discuss primary hypothyroidism.

Diet

Some studies suggest that a diet high in soy may decrease thyroid function. Natural-occurring chemicals in soy may interfere with the absorption of thyroid hormones that you may be taking. This is controversial in the medical literature, but if you are on a high soy diet, and you are suffering from a thyroid problem, then you may want to decrease or stop your soy intake to see if it improves your thyroid function.

Naturally occurring chemicals are contained in some vegetables that may disrupt normal function of the thyroid. Additionally, foods grown in nutritionally depleted soil may be deficient in important vitamins and minerals. (See related sections on nutritional deficiencies that follow.)

Iodine Deficiency

Iodine deficiency is a major cause of hypothyroidism and is the most common cause of hypothyroidism on a worldwide basis. Worldwide about one billion people are estimated to be iodine-deficient; however, it is unknown how often this results in hypothyroidism.

Iodine has therapeutic actions in the body. It is an antibacterial, anticancer, antiparasitic, antiviral, and mucolytic agent. The thyroid gland uses iodine on a daily basis. Iodine deficiency may affect other organs in the body as well, such as the kidneys, breasts, and prostate.

There are many causes of iodine deficiency, including the following:

- Food grown in iodine-depleted soil

- Diets without ocean fish or sea vegetables such as seaweed

- Inadequate use of iodized salt (low-salt diet) in a region such as the Midwest, which is low in iodine

The Importance of Iodine

Iodine is essential for everyone. It is a chemical element that is crucial for good health. Many conditions beside hypothyroidism may be improved with iodine supplementation, including:

- Dupuytren's contracture
- Excess mucous production
- Fatigue
- Fibrocystic breast disease
- Headaches/migraine headaches
- Hemorrhoids
- Keloids
- Ovarian cysts
- Parotid duct stones
- Peyronie's disease
- Sebaceous cysts

Moreover, breast health is related to iodine levels. Studies have shown that areas of the world with high iodine intake, like Japan, have a lower rate of breast cancer.

According to the World Health Organization, up to 72 percent of the world's population is affected by an iodine deficiency disorder. If you take thyroid hormone and you then start taking iodine, you may need less thyroid medication, therefore it is best if you have your iodine levels measured before you start on thyroid hormone. In fact, sometimes your symptoms of hypothyroidism may resolve, and your labs may normalize with just taking iodine if you are low in this important nutrient. Most people do better when they take iodine supplements to take both iodine and iodide as one preparation. Lugol's solution would be one way of doing this. It is a liquid but has a metallic taste so you may opt to take the iodine/iodine supplement as a pill.

- Diet that is high in pasta and breads, which contain bromide (bromide binds to iodine receptors and prevents iodine from binding)

- Fluoride use (inhibits iodine binding)

- Vegan and vegetarian diets

- Sucralose (artificial sweetener that contains chlorinated table sugar)

- Medications (the following are some examples, but any medication that contains bromide or fluoride can lead to iodine deficiency)

  o Atrovent inhaler (contains bromide)

  o Ipratropium nasal spray (contains bromide)

  o Pro-panthine (contains bromide)

  o Flonase (contains fluoride)

  o Flovent (contains fluoride)

If you are on one of these medications do not discontinue their use. Instead see your healthcare provider and have your iodine levels measured to see if you are deficient in iodine. Then your physician can make appropriate recommendations.

It is very important that you have your iodine levels measured before you start taking iodine. It is also important to take iodine when your levels are low. In mild-to-moderate iodine deficiency, increased thyroid activity can compensate for low iodine intake and maintain normal thyroid function in most individuals, but at a price: Chronic thyroid stimulation results in an increase in the prevalence of toxic nodular goiter and hyperthyroidism.

On the other hand, too much iodine in the diet, or by supplementation, has been associated with thyroiditis, which is an inflammation of your thyroid gland. High levels of iodine can cause it to be trapped by thyroglobulin. Elevated levels of iodinated thyroglobulin then prompt the immune system to react and to cause inflammation. Furthermore, research has shown that in some areas of the world where there is high dietary iodine content or excessive supplementation there is also an increase in not just thyroiditis but also thyroid cancer.

Therefore, it is important that you have your iodine levels measured before you begin iodine replacement. If you are on an iodine supplement, taking vitamin B_2 (riboflavin) and vitamin B_3 (niacin) helps make the iodine easier for the thyroid gland to absorb. Some studies suggest that if you have Hashimoto's thyroiditis (see page 55), then you should not supplement with iodine. More research needs to be done on this subject.

Iron Deficiency

One of the issues that may result from of an underactive thyroid is iron deficiency. In order for your thyroid to function optimally you have to have enough iron in your body. When the thyroid is underactive, the red blood cell production drops. Iron also plays a part in T4 to T3 conversion. In addition, iron is necessary for optimal immune system health, which is important if you are suffering from Graves' disease or Hashimoto's thyroiditis. Iron deficiency can be caused by the following:

- Loss of blood
- Consuming too little iron in your diet
- The body's inability to absorb iron
- For women, pregnancy and blood loss during the menstrual cycle. Consequently, women are more likely to be deficient in iron, especially in their childbearing years.
- Medications
- Proton-pump inhibitors like lansoprazole and omeprazole
- Antacids
- Ulcer medications like cimetidine and ranitidine

Magnesium Deficiency

Magnesium, the second most abundant intracellular cation (a positively charged ion), has been identified as a cofactor in over 300 enzymatic reactions involving energy metabolism, and protein and nucleic acid synthesis. Unfortunately, seven out of every ten Americans suffer from magnesium deficiency. Although there are several symptoms that may result from magnesium deficiency, the most common one is low thyroid function. Magnesium is necessary for the proper absorption of iodine. In addition, although magnesium is essential to every organ in your body, it is particularly important in the function of the heart, kidneys, and muscles. Magnesium deficiency can result when you take large doses of vitamin C. The problem being that vitamin C competes with magnesium. In addition, healthy thyroid function relies on a balance of calcium and magnesium in the body.

Other causes of magnesium deficiency include:

- Alcohol abuse
- Certain medications
- Diarrhea
- Eating a diet high in trans fatty acids
- Excessive sugar intake
- Extreme athletic competition
- Gastrointestinal disorders
- High caffeine intake
- Minimal intake of foods rich in magnesium
- Increased consumption of foods and drinks high in oxalic acid (such as almonds, cocoa, spinach, and tea)
- Phosphates in soft drinks
- Poor absorption
- Stress
- Surgery
- Taking magnesium supplements while eating a high-fiber meal
- Trauma

Selenium Deficiency

The mineral selenium is very important for your general health, as well as for your thyroid gland and thyroid hormones to function properly in your body. A deficiency in selenium can affect the conversion process of T4 to T3. Selenium deficiency can be rare, however it can develop under certain conditions. The following are some of these circumstances:

- Foods that are grown on poor selenium soils
- HIV
- Malabsorption, especially in the very elderly
- Severe gastrointestinal disorders such as Crohn's disease
- Surgery: small bowel resection, weight loss surgery
- Undergoing dialysis

Vitamin B Deficiency

A deficiency in vitamin B_2 can contribute to a low functioning thyroid. A lack of vitamin B_2 suppresses the production of T4 and keeps the thyroid and adrenal glands from secreting their hormones. Vitamin B_3 is needed to keep the endocrine cells in efficient working order. It plays a role in the production of thyroid hormones. Vitamin B₃ is needed to produce tyrosine (an amino acid) in the body, and T3 and T4 are derived from tyrosine. Also, be aware that taking vitamin B2 (riboflavin) and vitamin B₃ (niacin) is crucial if you are on iodine supplementation. It is also important in maintaining a healthy thyroid.

Vitamin D Deficiency

Like magnesium, many people are not aware that they have low levels of Vitamin D. Anyone can have vitamin D deficiency, including infants, children, and adults. Low levels of Vitamin D may interfere with the thyroid functioning properly. If you are suffering from an autoimmune thyroid condition, you can benefit from being tested for a deficiency in vitamin D. In addition, one of the most important roles of vitamin D is supporting immune health, which helps you ward off viruses and bacteria that cause illness. You can request your Vitamin D level to be checked when you have your next blood test. Besides taking daily vitamin D supplements, daily exposure to the sun is beneficial.

Zinc Deficiency

Without the existence of zinc in the body the thyroid cannot convert the less active hormone T4 to the active hormone T3. The hypothalamus also depends upon zinc to make the hormone it uses to cue the pituitary gland to switch on the thyroid. Too little zinc may lead to a low-functioning thyroid. In fact, zinc is a cofactor in over 100 reactions in the body. Chronic zinc deficiency can weaken your immune system.

Copper Deficiency

Optimal copper levels are needed to maintain thyroid function. Zinc and copper need to balance each other in the body: 10 to 15 mg of zinc to 1 mg of copper. Do not take copper supplements if you have Wilson's disease, a disorder that causes copper to accumulate in vital organs.

Medications, Nutrients, and Foods That Affect Thyroid Function and Use

Medications, nutrients, and/or foods are associated with a decrease in thyroid function and may affect how thyroid medication is used in the body. The mechanisms are numerous.

The following medications, nutrients, and foods interfere with thyroid medication absorption:

- Bile acid sequestrants (cholestyramine, colestipol, colesevelam)
- Calcium salts (carbonate, citrate, acetate)
- Cation exchange resins (Kayexalate)
- Charcoal
- Chromium picolinate
- Ciprofloxacin
- Ferrous sulfate
- H2 receptor antagonists
- Multivitamins (containing ferrous sulfate or calcium carbonate)
- Oral bisphosphonates
- Orlistat
- Phosphate binders (sevelamer, aluminum hydroxide)
- Proton pump inhibitors
- Raloxifene
- Sucralfate

The following increase clearance of thyroid hormone:

- Carbamazepine
- Growth hormone
- Nevirapine
- Oxcarbazepine
- Phenobarbital
- Phenytoin
- Primidone
- Quetiapine
- Rifampin
- Sertraline
- Stavudine
- Tyrosine kinase inhibitors (imatinib, sunitinib)

The conversion of T4 to T3 is inhibited by several drugs, including:

- Amiodarone
- Beta blockers (such as, propranolol and nadolol)
- Clomipramine
- Glucocorticoids
- Interleukin-6
- Iodinated contrast (ipodate, iopanoic acid)
- Ipodate
- Propylthiouracil

These drugs decrease the protein binding of levothyroxine:

- Carbamazepine
- Phenytoin

These medications reduce TSH concentration:

- Dopamine
- Octreotide
- Glucocorticoids

The following have direct and indirect effects on the hypothalamic-pituitary-thyroid axis:

- TSH secretion
  - ○ Decrease TSH secretion
    - Bexarotene
    - Dopamine
    - Dopaminergic agonists (bromocriptine, cabergoline)
    - Glucocorticoids
    - Thyroid hormone analogues
    - Somatostatin analogues (octreotide, lanreotide)
    - Somatostatin
    - Metformin
    - Opiates (e.g., heroin)
    - Interleukin-6
  - ○ Increase TSH secretion
    - Dopamine receptor blockers (metoclopramide)
    - Hypoadrenalism
    - Interleukin 2
    - Amphetamine
    - Ritonavir
    - St. John's Wort

These drugs interfere with thyroid hormone synthesis:

- Lithium
- Iodine
- Sulfonamides
- Many drugs and medical conditions also affect thyroid binding globulin (TBG)

TBG, when elevated, will bind more thyroid hormone, decreasing the free hormone available in the blood, which leads to stimulation of TSH, and the production of more thyroid hormone. In this case, the total thyroid hormone level will be high. These medications and conditions increase TBG:

- 5-Flurouracil
- Capecitabine
- Clofibrate
- Estrogens

- Hepatitis
- Heroin and other opioids
- Inherited
- Methadone
- Mitotane

- Neonatal state
- Perphanazine
- Porphyria
- Pregnancy
- SERMs (tamoxifen) raloxifene

These drugs and conditions decrease TBG, which causes the circulating thyroid hormone in the body to be reduced:

- Anabolic steroids
- Androgens (dehydroepiandrosterone (DHEA), dehydroepiandrosterone-sulfate (DHEA-S), testosterone, and dihydrotestosterone (DHT))
- Glucocorticoids
- Hepatic (liver) failure

- Inherited
- L-Asparaginase
- Nephrosis (also called nephrotic syndrome, which is a kidney disease)
- Nicotinic acid
- Severe illness

These medications and nutrients are also thyroid-binding inhibitors:

- Carbamazepine
- Free fatty acids
- Furosemide
- Heparin

- NSAIDs (variable and transient)
- Phenytoin
- Salicylates

If you rely on treatment with thyroid hormone medicine, taking certain supplements, for example calcium or iron, at the same time as the thyroid medication may decrease the amount of thyroid medicine that is being absorbed. It is recommended that calcium and iron supplements should not be taken at the same time as thyroid hormone medication. In addition, the absorption of thyroid medication can be impaired by soybean, papaya, grapefruit, and grapefruit juice. Espresso coffee and a high-fiber diet also decrease absorption. For optimal thyroid absorption, do not take any nutrients, or eat any food, or intake any drinks one hour before or one hour after taking your thyroid medication.

SIGNS AND SYMPTOMS

Early diagnosis of hypothyroidism isn't always easy. Most people with an underactive thyroid aren't aware that they have this condition. They may suffer a number of symptoms without recognizing that the symptoms are thyroid-related or that there may be no symptoms early on in the disease process. Often, the healthcare provider may minimize or misdiagnose the symptoms. Clinical manifestations of hypothyroidism range from life threatening to no signs or symptoms. The signs and symptoms of hypothyroidism normally progress slowly, over months or years, and quite often they may be confused with other disorders. The following are signs and symptoms of hypothyroidism:

- Acne
- Agitation/irritability
- Allergies
- Anemia (normocytic)
- Anxiety/panic attacks
- Bladder and kidney infections
- Blepharospasm (eye twitching)
- Bradycardia (slow heart rate)
- Carpal tunnel syndrome
- Cholesterol levels that are high (hypercholesterolemia)
- Cognitive decline
- Cold hands and feet
- Cold intolerance
- Congestive heart failure
- Constipation
- Coronary heart disease/acute myocardial infarction (heart attack)
- Course facial features

- Decreased cardiac output
- Decreased sexual interest
- Delayed deep tendon reflexes
- Deposition of mucin (glycoprotein) in connective tissues
- Depression
- Dizziness/vertigo
- Downturned mouth
- Drooping eyelids
- Dry skin
- Dull facial expression
- Ear canal that is dry, scaly, and may itch
- Ear wax build-up in the ear canal (cerumen)
- Easy bruising
- Eating disorders
- Elbows that are rough and bumpy (keratosis)
- Endometriosis
- Erectile dysfunction

- "Fat pads" above the clavicles
- Fatigue
- Fibrocystic breast disease
- Fluid retention
- Gallstones
- Goiter
- Hair loss in the front and back of the head
- Hair loss in varying amounts from legs, axilla, and arms
- Hair that is sparse, coarse, and dry
- Headaches, including migraine headaches
- High cortisol levels
- High C-reactive protein (CRP)
- Hoarse, husky voice
- High homocysteine levels (hyperhomocysteinemia)
- High insulin level (hyperinsulinemia)
- High prolactin level
- High triglycerides
- Hypertension (high blood pressure)
- Hypoglycemia (low blood sugar)
- Impaired kidney function
- Inability to concentrate
- Increased appetite

- Increased LDL (bad cholesterol)
- Increased risk of developing asthma
- Increased risk of developing bipolar disorder
- Increased risk of developing schizoid or affective psychoses
- Increased creatinine kinase (indicative of muscle damage)
- Infertility
- Insomnia
- Joint stiffness (arthralgias)
- Lethargy (lack of energy and enthusiasm)
- Loss of eyelashes or eyelashes that are not as thick
- Loss of one-third of the eyebrows
- Low amplitude theta and delta brain waves
- Low blood pressure
- Low body temperature
- Macroglossia (enlarged tongue)
- Menstrual cycle pain
- Menstrual irregularities including abnormally heavy bleeding (menorrhagia)
- Mild elevation of liver enzymes
- Miscarriage
- Morning stiffness

- Muscle and joint pain
- Muscle cramps
- Muscle weakness
- Muscular pain (myalgia)
- Nails that are brittle, easily broken, ridged, striated, thickened nails
- Nocturia (need to get up and urinate in the middle of the night)
- Nutritional imbalances
- Osteoporosis (bone loss)
- Paresthesia (abnormal sensation of feeling burning, tingling, and itching)
- Pericardiac effusion (buildup of too much fluid in the double-layered saclike structure around the heart (pericardium)
- Periorbital edema (fluid build-up around the eyes)
- Pleural effusion (accumulation of excess fluid in the pleural space, which is the potential space that surrounds each lung)
- Poor circulation
- Poor night vision
- Premenstrual syndrome (PMS)
- Proteinuria (abnormal quantities of protein in the urine)
- Puffy face
- Reduced heart rate
- Rough, dry skin
- Shortness of breath
- Sleep apnea
- Slow movements
- Slow speech
- Swollen eyelids
- Swollen legs, feet, hands, and abdomen
- Tendency to develop allergies
- Tinnitus (ringing in the ears)
- Vitamin B_{12} deficiency
- Voice changes
- Weight gain
- Yellowish skin discoloration due to the inability to convert beta carotene into vitamin A

There are some conditions that may be or may not be signs and symptoms of hypothyroidism, such as growth hormone deficiency in children, retrograde uterus, vitiligo, skin cancer, dry eyes, TMJ, and teeth clenching. If you suffer from any one or a number of these health issues, and no root cause has been found to alleviate the problem, perhaps it's time to consider looking at how well your thyroid is functioning.

DIAGNOSIS

Early detection of hypothyroidism is not always easy. However, there are a number of steps you can take to discover if you are suffering from an underactive thyroid. This process can incorporate several factors, such as clinical evaluation and blood tests. In addition, since a thyroid condition or disease may encompass many factors, other tests may be administered as well, such as imaging tests and biopsies.

Self-Awareness

As you have seen on page 37, there are many signs and symptoms associated with the underproduction of thyroid hormones. A lack of these key chemicals can cause many health issues to occur. If you see that you suffer from a number of these problems, you can conduct a simple home test to see if there might be a possibility of your having this condition.

Home Testing

If you are experiencing specific signs or symptoms that indicate you may have an underactive thyroid (see page 37, you can administer a safe and simple home test (see inset on page 41). You can determine the possibility of any potential thyroid dysfunction on your own, at your home, by measuring your basal temperature. Although this test is obviously not an official diagnosis of a thyroid dysfunction, it can give you some indication that you need to follow up with your physician for further testing to be administered.

Consult With Your Doctor or Other Healthcare Provider

If you feel a problem does exist, it is very important that you see your healthcare provider for an evaluation of your thyroid gland; and that you have a complete workup done and not a partial workup. Make sure your healthcare provider orders the following thyroid studies: TSH, free T3, free T4, reverse T3, and thyroid antibodies.

Clinical Evaluation

Your physician will perform a complete physical exam of the gland, where he/she palpates your thyroid to determine if there are any lumps, nodules, growths (goiters), or masses. In addition, he/she will be checking the thyroid's size, and if it is solid and firmly fixed in place.

Simple Home Tests to Determine Whether You Have a Potential Problem

The thyroid gland can be thought of as the body's thermostat. The hormones produced by the thyroid play a role in keeping you warm. Some patients will have normal or even optimal levels of thyroid hormone, but they still will have symptoms of hypothyroidism. For these individuals it is important to get a basal body temperature, since keeping the body at its optimal temperature setting cannot be achieved when the thyroid is struggling.

By measuring your basal temperature, yourself at home, you can determine if you have a thyroid issue. A basal body temperature is the temperature taken underneath your arm.

1. Place a mercury type thermometer within reach before bedtime.

2. Shake it down until you reach 96 degrees Fahrenheit.

3. Before you arise in the morning as soon as you awake place the thermometer under your armpit for 1 minute.

4. You take your temperature for three consecutive days and record the temperature.

A normal temperature is 97.8 to 98.2 degrees Fahrenheit. If you have an underactive thyroid, your average temperature will be lower than 97.8 degrees Fahrenheit. If you are a menstruating woman, then take your temperature during your menstrual cycle.

Blood Tests

The blood test is the most common test and plays an important role in diagnosing thyroid disease and treating thyroid conditions. Several blood tests will be done in order to determine if you are suffering from hypothyroidism. Your physician will be evaluating your TSH, free T4, freeT3, rt3 (reverse T3), and thyroid antibodies (see Table 1.2 on page 18).

Thyroid binding globulin (TBG) can also be measured (see page 19). This is the amount of stored hormone. It is produced by the liver and is affected by illness, liver disease, and some medications. Sometimes estrogens can raise TBG, so this is another test that your doctor may order.

Your healthcare provider may also order thyroid releasing hormone (TRH) also called thyrotropin-releasing factor (TRF), which is a hormone that stimulates the release of thyroid stimulating hormone (TSH) and prolactin from the pituitary. (See page 19.)

Some people have an autoimmune process where their body is literally trying to attack its own thyroid gland and the body produces a normal amount of thyroid hormone or not enough thyroid hormone. This is called Hashimoto's thyroiditis. Your test results will reveal that your thyroid antibody levels are high. (See Table 1.2 on page 18.) Also see the next chapter for a major discussion concerning Hashimoto's thyroiditis.

Imaging Tests

Laboratory tests may not be enough to diagnosis thyroid dysfunction. Sometimes more tests are ordered. Imaging tests are administered for a diagnosis of various thyroid disorders. The following are other tests that may be performed:

- Iodine Uptake Scan: to measure the absorption of iodine in the thyroid.

- Thyroid Scan: a radioisotope is administered, usually given with the iodine uptake. Cells that do not absorb iodine will appear "cold (lighter on the scan)," a cell absorbing too much iodine will appear "hot (darker)."

- Thyroid Ultrasound: high frequency sound waves provide an image of the thyroid gland. It aids in performing fine need biopsies.

Fine Needle Aspiration (FNA)

Fine needle aspiration is a type of biopsy procedure that is commonly performed to detect or rule out cancer cells in the thyroid. It is commonly performed on swellings or lumps found in the thyroid. The fine needle aspiration can identify the type of cells contained in the abnormal tissue or fluid.

TREATMENT

There are several things to consider in looking at treatment for low thyroid function. You may benefit from detoxification of the liver or helping your gut stay healthy. You may have nutritional deficiencies and improving your nutritional status may improve your thyroid function. You may be taking a medication that causes your thyroid not to function as well as it could. This does not mean that you should stop your medication, but it does mean that certain medications may cause your thyroid not to function optimally, and you may have to replace a nutrient that is deplete due to a medication or you may have to take thyroid medication due to another drug that you are taking. Last, you may benefit from thyroid replacement as a medication.

Detoxification

Sometimes individuals with a thyroid problem do not need medication but would benefit from a quality detoxification program. There is evidence that elements in the environment and diet can lead to thyroid conditions. You can treat these thyroid problems by detoxing your thyroid. PCBs, dioxins, DDT, HCB (hexachlorobenzene), phthalates, and high levels of heavy metals, such as lead, arsenic, and mercury can cause dysfunction of your thyroid gland, affecting both the production and conversion of thyroid hormones. It is possible to measure levels of most of these toxins and then work on their removal. Cleaning out many of the toxins will not only address your thyroid symptoms, but it will give you an overall sense of well-being and good health. There are several methods of detoxification that may need to be implemented. First, a liver detoxification program may be beneficial. If you have never used detoxification supplements it may be wise to consult with a doctor first.

- Take a quality cleansing product (pharmaceutical grade liver detox program)

- Eat healthy and avoid refined foods, sugars, and junk food

- Drink purified water and avoid alcohol, sodas, and sugar drinks

- Be sure that you are eliminating the toxins

With any detoxification program you need to follow certain guidelines to make it most effective. After your first detoxification program it is recommended that you go through detoxification once a year. (See also "Diet" on page 45.)

Furthermore, since some of these toxins are heavy metals, your health-care provider may opt to treat you with chelation in order to remove the heavy metals from your system. Likewise, some of the toxins may require sauna therapy to help remove them from the body.

In addition, your GI tract may need to be detoxified. The 5R program (Remove, Replace, Reinoculate, Repair, and Rebalance) is an effective way to stabilize and treat gastrointestinal dysfunction and to further gastrointestinal health.

Remove: The first step is to remove anything that may negatively affect your GI tract. They may be pesticides, foods you are sensitive to or allergic to, environmental toxins, or physical or psychological stress. Moreover, the factor that needs to be removed may be a pathogen such as a "bad" bacteria, fungus, or parasite, which may require medications or nutrients to eradicate.

Replace: The next step is to replace important nutrients that your body may be deficient in such as digestive enzymes, bile acids, hydrochloric acid, intrinsic secretions, and fiber. Your healthcare provider will lead you to the right therapies.

Reinoculate: Reinoculate refers to re-introducing "good" bacteria into the gut to repopulate the GI tract including probiotics (beneficial bacteria), prebiotics (fuel to feed the good bacteria), or both. For example, common species of good bacteria include *Bifidobacteria, Lactobacillus*, and the probiotic yeast *Saccharomyces boulardii*. Yogurt, tempeh, and sauerkraut are also sources of microbes that may have probiotic effects. In addition, prebiotic foods that contain inulin, which is a fiber, will also help the probiotics have a favorable environment. Artichoke, garlic, onions, leeks, and chicory root are all good sources. Taking a prebiotic also may be suggested by your doctor or nutritionist.

Repair: Nutrients are important to repair the lining of your GI tract. Arginine, glutamine, zinc, tocopherols, carotenoids, vitamins A, C, and D, pantothenic acid, folate, antioxidants, and omega-3 fatty acids have been shown to be beneficial.

Rebalance: Improving your lifestyle to promote less stress and more enjoyment will help to maintain the health of your gut. Getting enough sleep and exercising three to four times a week will help balance your life. Stress reduction techniques such as prayer, meditation, deep breathing, yoga, tai chi, and acupuncture, along with adaptogenic and calming herbs, are also helpful.

Sometimes when the patient's GI tract health is improved by using the 5R program they no longer have symptoms of hypothyroidism, and their labs also normalize.

Diet

Your diet and the kinds of foods you consume can provide you with some of the nutrients needed for a healthy thyroid gland. Whether or not you need a nutrient supplement in addition to your diet can be determined by a blood test that can indicate where you have nutritional deficiencies. Fortunately, there are supplements, herbs, and nutrients that can boost the conversion of T4 to T3. The following may be considered:

- Ashwagandha (an herb)
- High protein diet
- Iodine
- Iron
- Melatonin
- Potassium
- Replacement of testosterone in men (decreases the concentration of thyroid binding globulin)
- Selenium
- Tyrosine (an amino acid)
- Vitamins A, B_2, E
- Zinc

Some studies have shown that a diet high in soy may decrease thyroid function. This is controversial in the medical literature, but if you are on a high soy diet then you may want to decrease your soy intake to see if it improves your thyroid function.

A diet consisting of processed foods and sodas leads to magnesium deficiency. Therefore, try and limit your intake. Foods that are rich in magnesium consist of nuts and seeds, legumes, meats, and grains, such as rice and oats.

Iron can be found in foods such as meat, fish, and poultry, and the iron found in these foods is absorbed easily. Plant based foods, such as nuts, vegetables, grains, and fruits are less absorbable. To keep your ferritin (a protein in the body that binds iron) levels at normal range it is crucial to either get enough iron from the foods you eat or from a supplement or from both.

To ensure that you are consuming a rich source of vitamin B_2 you should include meat, mushrooms, almonds, whole grains, and leafy green vegetables in your diet. Foods high in vitamin B_3 are chicken and turkey, beef, and pine nuts. Some dietary sources of vitamin D include fish liver oils, beef liver, egg, alfalfa, and mushrooms. The mineral zinc can be found in protein rich foods, such as meat, nuts, legumes, seafood, and whole grains.

If you have high or positive thyroid antibodies, then the best thing that you can do is to stop ingesting any gluten. The next best thing that you can do is to help your gastrointestinal tract (GI tract) be healthier. (See the next chapter.)

Supplementation

There are several nutritional supplements you can take to stabilize your thyroid gland and restore its function, such as iodine, magnesium, selenium, vitamin B, vitamin D, and zinc. A deficiency in any of these nutrients can negatively affect your health. Not everyone with hypothyroidism is deficient in the same nutrients, therefore it is necessary to be tested to diagnose what you may be deficient in. If you are deficient in basic nutrients, then starting a multivitamin may help your thyroid function improve.

Copper. Optimal copper levels are needed to maintain thyroid function. Zinc and copper need to balance each other in the body: 10 to 15 mg of zinc to one mg of copper. Do not take copper supplements if you have Wilson's disease, a disorder that causes copper to accumulate in vital organs.

Iodine. Iodine has therapeutic actions in the body. It is an antibacterial, anticancer, antiparasitic, antiviral, and mucolytic agent. The thyroid gland uses iodine on a daily basis. Iodine is needed to produce thyroid hormones.

Iron. Iron and other minerals play an important role in hormone synthesis. A large number of animal and human studies have found that, with or without anemia, nutritional iron deficiency can affect thyroid metabolism, reduce plasma total T4 and T3 levels, reduce peripheral T4 to T3 conversion, and increase TSH levels. Optimal levels of ferritin are 100 ng/ml for men and menopausal women. If you are a menstruating woman, then your ferritin levels should be at least 130 ng/ml since you lose iron every month when you menstruate. Ferritin is a blood protein that stores iron. High levels of ferritin increase your risk of heart disease, so ask your healthcare provider if you need to take iron.

Magnesium. Magnesium plays a central role in thyroid disease. Magnesium is related to the stabilization of the structure of nucleic acids and seems also involved in DNA replication, transcription, and repair. There is a direct link between magnesium and a healthy thyroid and heart related conditions, however, a magnesium deficiency is difficult to test for. Currently, the most accurate measurement is a RBC magnesium level, which is the magnesium in your red blood cells rather than the magnesium in the blood serum. You can boost your magnesium intake by eating a well-balanced diet, which includes dark leafy green vegetables, seeds, and nuts, and eliminating caffeine from your diet. If you are taking any medications, check with your healthcare provider to see if there may be a possible negative interaction.

Molybdenum. Molybdenum is an essential micronutrient. Many studies have found that molybdenum is related to thyroid metabolism. In addition, this nutrient can interact with thyroid hormone receptors to positively affect thyroid hormone levels.

Selenium. In the thyroid, selenium is required for its antioxidant function and for the metabolism of thyroid hormones. One study looked at patients that were critically ill and showed that supplementation with selenium normalized thyroid lab results. Adding one or two Brazil nuts or garlic to your diet every day can help to provide you with the needed selenium. You can get toxic with the use of selenium; therefore, see your doctor or other healthcare provider before starting high doses of this important mineral.

Vitamin B_2. Making sure you are getting enough vitamin B_2 is necessary in regulating thyroid enzymes and maintaining healthy thyroid function. Eating almonds, eggs in moderation, cashews, salmon, and broccoli help to boost your B_2 levels.

Vitamin B_3. Vitamin B_3 is instrumental in building a strong immune system, and the cause of an underactive thyroid has often been associated with a weak immune system. For a mild vitamin B_3 deficiency, 50 mg twice a day is recommended.

Vitamin D. Vitamin D is key in keeping your bones strong; however, research suggests that low levels of vitamin D may have an effect on the thyroid working properly, as well as your immune system. See your healthcare provider to have her vitamin D levels measured to determine your exact dose.

Zinc. Zinc is essential for human health and plays a role in gene expression, cell division and growth, and in a variety of enzymes involved in immune and reproductive functioning. Zinc supplementation has been shown to help with optimal thyroid hormone metabolism. Eating a healthy diet and zinc supplements can be taken to treat a zinc deficiency. Taking too much zinc can cause toxicity. Zinc deficiency in humans can result from a reduced dietary intake and an inadequate absorption of the mineral.

Thyroid Hormone Replacement Therapy

When you consider thyroid hormone replacement, it is important to look at how the thyroid hormone is metabolized in the body. The body requires about 50 mg per year of iodine. About 70 percent of the T4 secreted daily is deiodinated to yield T3 and reverse T3 in equal parts. Eighty percent of circulating T3 comes from the peripheral monodeionization of T4 at the thyrosol ring, which occurs in the liver, kidney, and other tissues. Circulating reverse T3 is made the same way. Thyroid hormone is also metabolized in other pathways. It can be conjugated with glucuronate or sulfate and then excreted in the bile or it can be decarboxylated. Twenty percent to 40 percent of T4 is subsequently eliminated in the stool.

Studies have shown that most patients do better, if they need thyroid replacement, to have both T3 and T4 replaced. One study of 89 patients with hypothyroidism that were previously treated with T4 alone was compared to a group of people with low thyroid function that were not treated with T4. The symptoms of the patients already on T4 were not any different from the people who were untreated. In fact, intracellular thyroid hormone receptors have a high affinity for T3. Ninety percent of the thyroid hormone molecules that bind with the receptors are T3 and 10 percent are T4. Other studies have verified that most individuals have less symptoms if they are prescribed both T3 and T4. In another study the lab results were not better, but the patients felt better if they took both T3 and T4. Current thinking is that 98 percent of patients need both T3 and T4 replaced and only 2 percent do well on T4 alone. Make sure you see a healthcare provider that is fellowship trained in Anti-Aging and Regenerative Medicine or certified in Personalized Medicine. These providers will go according to your lab results so that you receive an individualized approach to your thyroid replacement.

There are different ways to take thyroid hormone replacement. They are all a prescription. You can take T4 alone, take T3 alone, or take both T4 and T3, which are commonly prescribed as desiccated thyroid, porcine (from a pig). If you have Hashimoto's thyroiditis (see page 55), some studies in the medical literature suggest that porcine thyroid replacement may not be the best form to take. This problem can be solved by your doctor prescribing non-porcine thyroid hormone, which is compounded.

The following are common combined thyroid hormones that are available in North America as a prescription. Most of them are close to four parts T4 to one part T3:

- Armour Thyroid
- NP Thyroid
- Nature-Throid
- WP Thyroid

- Westhroid
- Adthyza
- Liotrix
- Thyrolar

Next are the most common prescription T4 available in North America. All are immediate release and may contain lactose, which can interfere with thyroid hormone absorption. Absorption can vary from 48 to 80 percent:

- Eltroxin
- Levothyroid

- Levoxyl
- Synthroid

Last are the most common T3 medications available in North America, all of, which are immediate release:

- Cytomel
- Triostat (injectable)

- Liothyronine sodium (generic)

Compounded thyroid medication is made by a compounding pharmacy that is specially trained to make compounded medications. The advantage to having your thyroid hormone compounded is that you then can have the ratio of your T4 to T3 be any ratio that you want it to be. Four to one may not be the best ratio for you. In other words, compounded prescription thyroid medication is customized to your own needs. It is personalized. One size does not fit all patients. Also, you are getting no fillers that are not needed and the physician who writes your prescription for compounded thyroid hormone can also add selenium, chromium, zinc, iodine, or other nutrients if this is something that you would like to do.

It is crucial that when you start on thyroid medication that you have your thyroid levels re-measured in six weeks. Once you have an optimal dosage schedule then your thyroid level should be measured again every six months. There are things that can change your dose of thyroid medication, such as weight gain or weight loss. The amount of stress that you have may also affect your thyroid dosage.

OUTCOME (PROGNOSIS)

Once the source of the hypothyroidism has been identified and elimi-nated, any further damage to the thyroid gland should stop. However, normally, patients are put on a combination of T3 and T4 hormone for the remainder of their lives to keep their thyroid levels optimal. Once done, all the symptoms and signs of hypothyroidism should be reversed.

Interestingly, there are situations where the body will produce normal TSH levels, however the patient may still have symptoms. Your health care provider will in this state of affairs consider the following differential diagnosis:

- Anemia (B_{12} or iron deficiency)

- Autoimmune disorders: adrenal insufficiency, atrophic gastritis with pernicious anemia, rheumatoid arthritis

- Chronic kidney disease

- Diabetes type I

- Liver disease

- Menopause

- Mental health disorders: depression, anxiety

- Obstructive sleep apnea

- Viral infections: mononucleosis, Lyme disease, HIV, COVID-19

Hypothyroidism and the Aging Process

Twenty years ago, a low serum TSH level was first associated with an increased risk of atrial fibrillation and other cardiovascular events, oste-oporotic fracture, dementia, and death. However, several studies have found an association of elevated serum TSH with adverse cardiac out-comes, including myocardial infarction (MI), heart failure, and mortality. In contrast, some authors have suggested that an elevated serum TSH in older age might have no adverse effect on health although one study of individuals 85 years and older showed that a high serum TSH at baseline was associated with a favorable outcome compared with that of other people in their age group. Consequently, it is suggested that for individ-uals over the age of 85 that the upper limit of normal TSH should be 2.5 to 3.0 and not 2.0. There is the perfect balance of thyroid medication for every patient, particularly as they age.

DISORDERS CAUSED BY OR ASSOCIATED WITH HYPOTHYROIDISM

There are many diseases and conditions that have been associated with hypothyroidism. Depression has been strongly associated with hypothyroidism, as have heart disease, and memory loss. These disease processes are covered in separate chapters in this book.

Ankylosing Spondylitis (AS)

Ankylosing spondylitis is a kind of chronic rheumatic disease that affects the spine. The spine's vertebrae may fuse together, causing pain and stiffness from the neck down to the lower back. Eventually it may result in a stooped-over posture. This condition affects men two to three times more commonly than women. The inflammation that occurs in ankylosing spondylitis has been a subject of research. This inflammatory process has been linked in some individuals with low-functioning thyroid and the activation of the body's immune system.

Attention Deficit Hyperactivity Disorder

Attention Deficit Hyperactivity Disorder is a condition characterized by impulsive symptoms, inattention, being easily distracted, forgetfulness, and hyperactivity that affects everyday functioning. Some studies have shown that ADHD may be related to thyroid dysfunction. They found that increased levels of TSH correlated with an inability to sustain one's attention.

Chronic Fatigue Syndrome (CFS)

Chronic fatigue syndrome has been associated with an underactive thyroid; however, it is very often misdiagnosed. When diagnosed properly, the majority of cases are women in the age bracket of 25 to 45 years old. CFS is a medical condition where you suffer from long-term fatigue that is not due to exertion and this condition puts limitations on your ability to carry out normal daily activities. Research has indicated that a relationship may exist between CFS and thyroid autoimmunity. These studies suggest that the immune system may be chronically active, which would explain the fatigue and lack of energy experienced with this disease.

Fibromyalgia (FMS)

Fibromyalgia is an arthritic related condition characterized by widespread musculoskeletal pain, soreness, and tenderness that rarely disappears. It is one of the most common chronic pain conditions and it also affects women more than men. The most common symptoms of FMS mimic low thyroid symptoms and are therefore often misdiagnosed. Some experts suggest that FMS is also related to immune dysfunction and others suggest that it is an indication of an underactive metabolism, a low thyroid disorder, and/or a dysfunction of the mitochondria (the energy producing cells of the body). Studies have recently revealed that there is a high prevalence of anti-TSH receptor antibodies in fibromyalgia syndrome.

Rosacea

Rosacea is a chronic inflammatory disease of the skin with an unknown cause. Erythematous papules and pustules and telangiectasia on the cheeks, nose, forehead, and occasionally around the eyes as well as irreversible chronic inflammation of nose, which leads to hypertrophy that is irreversible (rhinophyma). Intermittent flushing occurs in the affected area. Some people develop gut symptoms and others may have symptoms related to their eyes such as conjunctivitis, dry and burning eyes, corneal abnormalities, and blepharitis (eye spasming). Studies have revealed the rate of hypothyroidism was significantly increased in rosacea patients in both genders. The frequency of hypothyroidism was highest in the age range of 40 to 49. Hypothyroidism may be involved among the comorbidities of rosacea and investigation for hypothyroidism may be an appropriate approach when evaluating rosacea patients.

Meniere's Disease

Meniere's disease is also called idiopathic endolymphatic hydrops. This disease is characterized by excessive fluid in the ear, which causes recurrent episodes of tinnitus, vertigo, and hearing loss. People commonly complain of a feeling of pressure or fullness in the ear. Typically, only one ear is affected, however, over time both ears may become involved. Other symptoms may include anxiety, nausea, diarrhea, blurred vision, rapid pulse, cold sweats, and trembling. Attacks usually last 20 minutes for an entire day. Recurrence is variable from several times a week to several months apart. The individual may feel tired after the episode. Thyroid diseases of goiter, hypothyroidism, and hyperthyroidism have been found to be associated with Meniere's disease.

Migraine Headaches

Migraine headaches are caused by genetic susceptibility that is triggered by environmental as well as biological factors. Studies conducted on children, teens, and adults have shown an association between subclinical hypothyroidism and migraine headaches. In fact, in one study, the prevalence of lifetime migraine in individuals with subclinical hypothyroidism was significantly higher than controls (62 percent vs. 18 percent).

Hypertension

Hypothyroidism has been recognized as a cause of secondary hypertension. Previous studies on the prevalence of hypertension in individuals with hypothyroidism have demonstrated elevated blood pressure values. Increased peripheral vascular resistance and low cardiac output has been suggested to be the possible link between hypothyroidism and diastolic hypertension. The hypothyroid population is characterized by significant volume changes, initiating a volume-dependent, low plasma renin activity mechanism of blood pressure elevation. In addition, one study found that in patients with hypertension and hypothyroidism, 50 percent of patients had their hypertension completely reversed when prescribed thyroid hormone replacement therapy. This may be related to arterial stiffness, which is found in even subclinical cases of hypothyroidism.

Infertility

Some individuals with infertility and menstrual irregularities have underlying chronic thyroiditis in conjunction with subclinical or overt hypothyroidism. Moreover, TPOAb-positive people, even with normal thyroid function, have an excess miscarriage rate. Typically, these individuals go to their healthcare provider because of infertility or a previous miscarriage, rather than hypothyroidism. A careful evaluation may identify chronic thyroiditis. Furthermore, in some patients with hypothyroidism, thyroid hormone replacement therapy may normalize the menstrual cycle and restore normal fertility.

CONCLUSION

Given that thyroid hormone receptors are present in nearly all tissues, hypothyroidism may have pervasive effects on multiple end-organs (e.g., neuropsychiatric, hematologic, musculoskeletal). Optimal thyroid function requires adequate nutritional intake. It is also related to toxin exposure, other hormonal function and dysfunction, and medication usage. Likewise, as you have seen in this chapter, many factors determine perfect thyroid function, including accurate measuring techniques. Most individuals that require thyroid replacement benefit from both T3 and T4 to optimize thyroid function and consequently improve overall health. In the next chapter you will learn more about Hashimoto's thyroiditis, a condition that commonly is associated with hypothyroidism.

3

Hashimoto's Thyroiditis (HT)

Hashimoto's thyroiditis (HT), also called Hashimoto's disease, chronic lymphocytic thyroiditis, and autoimmune thyroiditis, is an autoimmune condition in, which the thyroid gland is gradually destroyed. It was first described by the Japanese physician Hakaru Hashimoto in 1912. As the tissues of the gland become inflamed, the thyroid produces less hormones, interfering with the body's normal metabolism. The disease begins slowly and may go undetected for months or even years. It is the most common cause of hypothyroidism in the United States and other countries where iodine deficiency is less common.

Autoimmune thyroid diseases (AITDs) have been estimated to be 5 to 10 times more common in women than in men. AITDs are characterized pathologically by infiltration of the thyroid with sensitized T lymphocytes and serologically by circulating thyroid autoantibodies. Autoimmunity to the thyroid gland appears to be an inherited defect in immune surveillance, leading to abnormal regulation of immune responsiveness or alteration of presenting antigen in the thyroid. One of the keys to diagnosing AITDs is determining the presence of elevated anti-thyroid antibody titers, which include anti-thyroglobulin antibodies (TgAb), anti–microsomal/thyroid peroxidase antibodies (TPOAb), and TSH receptor antibodies (TSHRAb). Many patients with chronic autoimmune thyroiditis are biochemically euthyroid (have a normal functioning thyroid gland). However, approximately 75 percent have elevated anti-thyroid antibody titers. Once present, these antibodies generally persist, with spontaneous disappearance occurring infrequently. Among the disease-free population in the NHANES survey, tests for TgAb were positive in 10.4 percent and TPOAb in 11.3 percent. These antibodies were more common in women than men and increased with age. Only positive TPOAb tests were significantly associated with hypothyroidism. The presence of elevated TPOAb titers in patients with subclinical hypothyroidism helps to predict progression to overt hypothyroidism—4.3 percent per year with TPOAb vs. 2.6 percent per year without elevated TPOAb titers.

Generally, the symptoms and signs resemble those of hypothyroidism. The disease progresses slowly and causes a chronic thyroid disorder.

Not surprisingly, there is also an increased frequency of other auto-immune disorders in people with Hashimoto's thyroiditis such as type 1 diabetes, pernicious anemia, primary adrenal failure (Addison's disease), myasthenia gravis, celiac disease, rheumatoid arthritis, systemic lupus erythematosus (SLE), and rarely thyroid lymphoma.

RISK FACTORS

The flare-up of antibodies that are at the root cause of Hashimoto's thyroiditis can be initiated for any number of reasons. The following factors may indicate if an individual is at a higher risk.

Age

The signs of Hashimoto's thyroiditis usually present between the ages of 30 and 50. The disease can occur in children, teens, and young women.

Gender

As with most thyroid related diseases, women are more prone to develop HT than men.

Genetics

Recent research has shown a significant role of heredity in the development of autoimmune thyroid disease or Hashimoto's thyroiditis. In addition, other autoimmune prone genes may trigger this condition as well. However, it may require one or more environmental factors, as listed below, to initiate this condition.

CAUSES

There are several conditions that may trigger Hashimoto's thyroiditis. These include the following.

Environmental Exposure

There are a number of chemicals that may lead to the development of HT as well as other forms of autoimmune diseases. These include perchlorate, fluoride, lithium, mercury, bisphenol A, and Teflon.

Smoking

Smoking was found to be associated with lower levels of total T4 in women.

Excessive Iodine

A diet heavy in foods containing iodine, taking iodine supplements, and/ or taking drugs containing large amounts of iodine can trigger HT. In addition, the introduction of universal salt iodization can have a similar, although transient effect.

Helicobacter pylori (H. pylori)

H. pylori infection in the stomach has been proposed to imitate the antigenic components of the thyroid cell membrane and may play a leading role in the onset of autoimmune diseases, such as Hashimoto's thyroiditis.

Pregnancy

Pregnancy creates great hormonal changes in a woman's body. Sometimes this can result in some form of thyroid dysfunction during or after pregnancy. Statistics indicate that approximately 20 percent of the women who have thyroid issues during pregnancy will develop HT in later years.

Radiation Exposure

While less common, research has shown that being exposed to large amounts of radiation can bring on autoimmune thyroid diseases.

Inflammation

A downregulation of suppressor T-lymphocytes and the ensuing activity against thyroglobulin (TgAb) and thyroid-peroxidase (TPOAb), one essential for the production and storage of thyroid hormones and the other involved in hormone synthesis, respectively, appear to be the starting point of the autoimmune process. Once the inflammatory cascade has been activated and the mechanism initiated, T-lymphocytes may trigger a production of specific antibodies by B-lymphocytes. Therefore, autoreactive B lymphocytes play a specific role in the induction of Hashimoto's thyroiditis.

Oxidative Stress

Oxidative stress has been shown to be responsible for the onset of these autoimmunity disorders. Oxidative stress is an imbalance between the production of free radicals and the ability of the body to counteract or detoxify their harmful effects through neutralization by antioxidants. A free radical is an oxygen containing molecule that has one or more unpaired electrons, making it highly reactive with other molecules. Hence, an increase of TPOAb and TgAb concentration is largely seen. The concentration of these antibodies, as well as thyroid morphology, and the ability of follicular cells to produce thyroid hormones may change during life. Their presence may cause continuous damage to the thyroid tissue, leading to a decrease in hormone production.

SIGNS AND SYMPTOMS

The signs and symptoms of Hashimoto's thyroiditis are the same as those for hypothyroidism. Early diagnosis of hypothyroidism isn't always easy. Most people with an underactive thyroid aren't aware that they have this condition. They may suffer from one or many symptoms without recognizing that the symptoms are thyroid-related or that there may be no symptoms early on in the disease process. Often, a healthcare provider may minimize or misdiagnose the symptoms. The signs and symptoms of hypothyroidism normally progress slowly, over months or years, and quite often they may be confused with other disorders. The following are some of the signs and symptoms of hypothyroidism:

- Acne
- Agitation/irritability
- Allergies
- Anxiety/panic attacks
- Arrhythmias (irregular heart rhythm)
- Bladder and kidney infections
- Blepharospasm (eye twitching) is more common
- Carpal tunnel syndrome
- Cholesterol levels that are high (hypercholesterolemia)
- Cognitive decline
- Cold hands and feet

- Cold intolerance
- Congestive heart failure
- Constipation
- Coronary heart disease/acute myocardial infarction (heart attack)
- Decreased cardiac output
- Decreased sexual interest
- Delayed deep tendon reflexes
- Deposition of mucin (glycoprotein) in connective tissues
- Depression
- Dizziness/vertigo
- Downturned mouth
- Drooping eyelids
- Dull facial expression
- Ear canal that is dry, scaly, and may itch
- Ear wax build-up in the ear canal (cerumen)
- Easy bruising
- Eating disorders
- Elbows that are rough and bumpy (keratosis)
- Endometriosis
- Erectile dysfunction
- "Fat pads" above the clavicles
- Fatigue
- Fibrocystic breast disease
- Fluid retention
- Gallstones

- Hair loss in the front and back of the head
- Hair loss in varying amounts from legs, axilla, and arms
- Hair that is sparse, coarse, and dry
- Headaches, including migraine headaches
- High cortisol levels
- High C-reactive protein (CRP)
- Hoarse, husky voice
- High homocysteine levels (hyperhomocysteinemia)
- High insulin levels (hyperinsulinemia)
- Hypertension (high blood pressure)
- Hypoglycemia (low blood sugar)
- Impaired kidney function
- Inability to concentrate
- Increased appetite
- Increased risk of developing asthma
- Increased risk of developing bipolar disorder
- Increased risk of developing schizoid or affective psychoses
- Infertility
- Insomnia
- Iron deficiency anemia
- Joint stiffness (arthralgias)

- Loss of eyelashes or eyelashes that are not as thick
- Loss of one-third of the eyebrows
- Low amplitude theta and delta brain waves.
- Low blood pressure
- Low body temperature
- Menstrual cycle pain
- Menstrual irregularities including abnormally heavy bleeding
- Mild elevation of liver enzymes
- Miscarriage
- Morning stiffness
- Muscle and joint pain
- Muscle craps
- Muscle weakness
- Muscular pain
- Nails that are brittle, easily broken, ridged, striated, thickened nails
- Nocturia (need to get up and urinate in the middle of the night)
- Nutritional imbalances
- Osteoporosis (bone loss)
- Paresthesia (abnormal sensation of feeling burning, tingling, and itching)
- Poor circulation
- Poor night vision
- Premenstrual syndrome (PMS)
- Puffy face
- Reduced heart rate
- Rough, dry skin
- Shortness of breath
- Sleep apnea
- Slow movements
- Slow speech
- Swollen eyelids
- Swollen legs, feet, hands, and abdomen
- Tendency to develop allergies
- Tinnitus (ringing in the ears)
- Vitamin B_{12} deficiency
- Weight gain
- Yellowish skin discoloration due to the inability to convert beta carotene into vitamin A

There are some conditions that may or may not be signs and symptoms of hypothyroidism, such as growth hormone deficiency in children, retrograde uterus, vitiligo, skin cancer, dry eyes, TMJ, and teeth clenching. If you suffer from any one or a number of these health issues, and no root cause has been found to alleviate the problem, perhaps it's time to consider looking at how well your thyroid is functioning.

DIAGNOSIS

Early diagnosis of Hashimoto's thyroiditis isn't always easy. As previously mentioned, people with an underactive thyroid aren't always aware that they have this condition. They may suffer a number of symptoms without realizing they have a thyroid problem. There are several tests to indicate whether or not it may be Hashimoto's thyroiditis. The key factor is to determine if the hypothyroidism is being caused by an autoimmune reaction. This requires your practitioner measuring thyroid antibodies. Many healthcare providers only measure TSH or TSH and free T4.

Self-Awareness

As you have seen on page 37, there are many signs and symptoms associated with the underproduction of thyroid hormones. Low levels of thyroid hormones can cause many health issues to occur. If you see that you suffer from a number of these problems, you can conduct a simple home test to see if there might be a possibility of your having this condition.

Home Testing

If you are experiencing specific signs or symptoms that indicate you may have an underactive thyroid (see page 37), you can administer a safe and simple home test (see inset on page 41). You can determine the possibility of any potential thyroid dysfunction on your own, at your home, by measuring your basal temperature. Although this test is obviously not an official diagnosis of a thyroid dysfunction, it can give you some indication that you need to follow up with your physician for further testing to be administered.

Consult With Your Doctor or Other Healthcare Provider

If you feel a problem does exist, it is very important that you see your healthcare provider for an evaluation of your thyroid gland, and that you have a complete workup done and not a partial workup.

Clinical Evaluation

Your physician will perform a complete physical exam of the gland, where he/she palpates your thyroid to determine if there are any lumps, nodules, growths (goiters), or masses. In addition, he/she will be checking the thyroid's size, and if it is solid and firmly fixed in place.

Blood Tests

The blood test is the most common test and plays an important role in diagnosing thyroid disease and treating thyroid conditions. A few blood tests will be done in order to determine if you are suffering from hypothyroidism. Your physician will be evaluating your TSH, free T4, freeT3, rt3 (reverse T3), and thyroid antibodies (see Table 1.2 on page 18).

Thyroid Binding Globulin (TBG). Thyroid binding globulin (TBG) can also be measured (see page 19). This is the amount of stored hormone. It is produced by the liver and is affected by illness, liver disease, and some medications. Sometimes estrogens can raise TBG, so this is another test that your doctor may order.

Thyroid Releasing Hormone (TRH). Your healthcare provider may also order thyroid releasing hormone (TRH), also called thyrotropin-releasing factor (TRF), which is a hormone that stimulates the release of thyroid stimulating hormone (TSH) and prolactin from the pituitary (see page 20).

In addition, with Hashimoto's thyroiditis, high antibody level compared to a lowered level of thyroid hormones will indicate the presence of autoimmune problem. Likewise, it is not as common, but you can have normal levels of TSH, free T3, and free T4 with positive antibodies and you would still have Hashimoto's thyroiditis.

Fine Needle Aspiration (FNA)

Fine needle aspiration is a type of biopsy procedure that is commonly performed to detect or rule out cancer cells in the thyroid. It is commonly performed on swellings or lumps found in the thyroid. The fine needle aspiration can identify the type of cells contained in the abnormal tissue or fluid.

Imaging Tests

Laboratory tests may not be enough to diagnosis thyroid dysfunction. Sometimes more tests are ordered. Imaging tests are administered for a diagnosis of various thyroid disorders. The following are some other tests that may be performed:

- Iodine Uptake Scan: to measure the absorption of iodine in the thyroid.

- Thyroid Scan: a radioisotope is administered, usually given with the iodine uptake. Cells that do not absorb iodine will appear "cold" (lighter on the scan), a cell absorbing too much iodine will appear "hot" (darker).

- Thyroid Ultrasound: high frequency sound waves provide an image of the thyroid gland. It aids in performing fine need biopsies.

TREATMENT OF HASHIMOTO'S THYROIDITIS WITH NORMAL THYROID FUNCTION

Ten to twenty percent of individuals with Hashimoto's thyroiditis have normal thyroid function. Therefore, the treatment is centered around decreasing the autoimmune response. Since HT is an autoimmune process, the suggested therapy is to avoid all gluten as a life-long change. Furthermore, when you have an autoimmune disorder, your GI tract (gut) is not healthy. Have your healthcare provider order a functional medicine GI function test and any imbalance will be treated according to the lab results. After your GI tract is healthy, discuss with your doctor starting the medication low-dose naltrexone (LDN) to decrease the inflammatory response that occurs in Hashimoto's. (See page 70.)

TREATMENT OF HASHIMOTO'S THYROIDITIS WITH HYPOTHYROIDISM

There are several things to consider in looking at treatment for low thyroid function. You may benefit from detoxification of the liver or helping your gut stay healthy. You may have nutritional deficiencies and improving your nutritional status may improve your thyroid function. You may be taking a medication that causes your thyroid not to function as well as it could. This does not mean that you should stop your medication, but it does mean that certain medications may cause your thyroid not to function optimally, and you may have to replace a nutrient that is deplete due to a medication or you may have to take thyroid medication due to another drug that you are taking. Last, in general, you may benefit from thyroid replacement as a medication.

Detoxification

Sometimes individuals with a thyroid problem do not need medication but would benefit from a quality detoxification program. There is evidence that elements in the environment and diet can lead to thyroid conditions. You can treat these thyroid problems by detoxing your thyroid. PCBs, dioxins, DDT, HCB (hexachlorobenzene), phthalates, and high levels of heavy metals, such as lead, arsenic, and mercury can cause dysfunction of your thyroid gland, affecting both the production and conversion of thyroid hormones. It is possible to measure levels of most of these toxins and then work on their removal. Cleaning out many of the toxins will not only address your thyroid symptoms, but it will give you an overall sense of well-being and good health.

There are several methods of detoxification that may need to be implemented. First, a liver detoxification program may be beneficial. If you have never used detoxification supplements it may be wise to consult with a doctor first.

- Take a quality cleansing product
- Eat healthy and avoid refined foods, sugars, and junk food
- Drink purified water and avoid alcohol, sodas, and sugar drinks
- Be sure that you are eliminating the toxins

With any detoxification program you need to follow certain guidelines to make it most effective. After your first detoxification program it is recommended that you go through detoxification once a year. (See also "Diet" on page 65.)

Since some of these toxins are heavy metals, your healthcare provider may opt to treat you with a chelation agent in order to remove the heavy metals from your system. Some of the toxins may require sauna therapy to help remove them from the body.

In addition, your GI tract may need to be detoxified. The 5R program (Remove, Replace, Reinoculate, Repair, and Rebalance) is an effective way to stabilize and treat gastrointestinal dysfunction and to further gastrointestinal health.

Remove: The first step is to remove anything that may negatively affect your GI tract. They may be pesticides, foods you are sensitive to or allergic to, environmental toxins, or physical or psychological stress. Moreover, the factor that needs to be removed may be a pathogen such as a "bad" bacteria, fungus, or parasite, which may require medications or nutrients to eradicate.

Replace: The next step is to replace important nutrients that your body may be deficient in such as digestive enzymes, bile acids, hydrochloric acid, intrinsic secretions, and/or fiber. Your healthcare provider will lead you to the right therapies.

Reinoculate: Reinoculate refers to re-introducing "good" bacteria into the gut to repopulate the GI tract including probiotics (beneficial bacteria), prebiotics (fuel to feed the good bacteria), or both. For example, common species of good bacteria include *Bifidobacteria, Lactobacillus,* and the probiotic yeast *Saccharomyces boulardii.* Yogurt, tempeh, and sauerkraut are also sources of microbes, which may have probiotic effects. In addition, prebiotic foods that contain inulin, which is a fiber, will also help the probiotics have a favorable environment. Artichoke, garlic, onions, leeks, and chicory root are all good sources. Taking a prebiotic, moreover, also may be suggested by your doctor or nutritionist.

Repair: Nutrients are important to repair the lining of your GI tract. Arginine, glutamine, zinc, tocopherols, carotenoids, vitamins A, C, and D, pantothenic acid, folate, antioxidants, and omega-3 fatty acids have been shown to be beneficial.

Rebalance: Improving your lifestyle to promote less stress and more enjoyment will help to maintain the health of your gut. Getting enough sleep and exercising three to four times a week will help balance your life. Stress reduction techniques such as prayer, meditation, deep breathing, yoga, tai chi, and acupuncture, along with adaptogenic and calming herbs, are also helpful.

Sometimes when the patient's GI tract health is improved by using the 5R program they no longer have symptoms of hypothyroidism, and their labs also normalize including their antibodies.

Diet

It is very important if you have Hashimoto's thyroiditis that you avoid all gluten as a life-long change due to the interactions of gliadin with thyroid antigens. You should also consider eliminating lactose (milk products with lactose) because of intolerance and interactions with thyroid medication. Observational and controlled trials have shown frequent nutrition deficiencies in HT patients. Your diet and the kinds of foods you consume can provide you with some of the nutrients needed for a healthy thyroid gland. Whether or not you need a nutrient supplement, in addition to your diet, can be determined by a blood test that will indicate where you are deficient. Fortunately, there are supplements, herbs, and nutrients that can boost the conversion of T4 to T3. The following may be considered:

- Ashwagandha (an herb)
- High protein diet
- Iodine
- Iron
- Melatonin
- Potassium

- Replacement of testosterone in men (decreases the concentration of thyroid binding globulin)
- Selenium
- Tyrosine (an amino acid)
- Vitamins A, B_2, E
- Zinc

Some studies have shown that a diet high in soy may decrease thyroid function. This is controversial in the medical literature, but if you are on a high soy diet then you may want to decrease your soy intake to see if it improves your thyroid function.

A diet consisting of processed foods and sodas leads to magnesium deficiency. Foods that are rich in magnesium consist of nuts and seeds, legumes, meats, and grains, such as rice and oats.

Iron can be found in foods such as meat, fish, and poultry, and the iron found in these foods is absorbed easily. Plant based foods, such as nuts, vegetables, grains, and fruits, are less absorbable. To keep your ferritin (a protein in the body that binds iron) levels at normal range it is crucial to either get enough iron from the foods you eat, or from a supplement, or from both.

To ensure that you are consuming a rich source of vitamin B_2 you should include meat, mushrooms, almonds, whole grains, and leafy green vegetables in your diet. Foods high in vitamin B_3 are chicken and turkey, beef, and pine nuts. Some dietary sources of vitamin D include fish liver oils, beef liver, egg, alfalfa, and mushrooms. The mineral zinc can be found in protein rich foods, such as meat, nuts, legumes, seafood, and whole grains.

If you have high or positive thyroid antibodies, then the best thing that you can do related to your diet is to stop ingesting any gluten. In addition, the role of the proper level of protein intake and dietary fiber are beneficial. Moreover, the regulation of the immune system by an anti-inflammatory diet is helpful. Foods such as berries (strawberries, blueberries, raspberries, and blackberries), fatty fish such as salmon, broccoli, avocados, tomatoes, cherries, and even dark chocolate are anti-inflammatory, as is extra virgin olive oil, and turmeric.

Supplementation

There are nutritional supplements you can take to stabilize your thyroid gland and restore its function, such as iodine, magnesium, selenium, vitamin B, vitamin D, and zinc. A deficiency in any of these nutrients can negatively affect your health. Not everyone with Hashimoto's is low in the same nutrients, therefore it is necessary to be tested to diagnose what you may be deficient in. If you are deficient in basic nutrients, then starting a multivitamin may help your thyroid function improve.

In addition, studies have shown that oxidants are increased, and anti-oxidants are decreased in patients with euthyroid autoimmune thyroiditis, and that oxidative/anti-oxidative balance is shifted to the oxidative side as previously mentioned. Therefore, increased oxidative stress may have a role in thyroid autoimmunity. Consequently, the need for more antioxidants is greater in Hashimoto's thyroiditis than it is in individuals with hypothyroidism that is not autoimmune related.

Copper. Optimal copper levels are needed to maintain thyroid function. Zinc and copper need to balance each other in the body: 10 to 15 mg of zinc to 1 mg of copper. Do not take copper supplements if you have Wilson's disease, a disorder that causes copper to accumulate in vital organs.

Inositol. In a study of 86 patients with Hashimoto's thyroiditis and subclinical hypothyroidism, the authors found that the administration of myo-inositol and selenomethionine for six months significantly decreased TSH, TPOAb, and TgAb concentrations, while at the same time enhancing thyroid hormones and personal well-being, thereby restoring normal thyroid levels in patients diagnosed with autoimmune thyroiditis. Therefore, it can be speculated that impairment of the inositol-dependent TSH signaling pathway may be, at least in part, one cause of thyroid malfunctioning and that, by increasing the availability of myo-inositol at the cellular level, it is possible to improve TSH sensitivity of the thyroid follicular cell. In fact, previous clinical studies, as well as this one, indicate that the administration of 600 mg myo-inositol is able to ameliorate thyroid function and symptomatology in patients with Hashimoto's thyroiditis.

Iodine. Iodine has therapeutic actions in the body. It is an antibacterial, anticancer, antiparasitic, antiviral, and mucolytic agent. The thyroid gland uses iodine on a daily basis. Iodine is needed for the production of thyroid hormones. High iodine intakes are well tolerated by most healthy individuals, but in some people, excess iodine intakes may precipitate hyperthyroidism, hypothyroidism, goiter, and/or thyroid autoimmunity.

Iron. Iron and other minerals play an important role in hormone synthesis. A large number of animal and human studies have found that, with or without anemia, nutritional iron deficiency can affect thyroid metabolism, reduce plasma total T4 and T3 levels, reduce peripheral T4 to T3 conversion, and increase TSH levels. Optimal levels of ferritin (storage iron) are 100 ng/ml. If you are a menstruating woman then your ferritin levels should be at least 130 ng/ml since you lose iron every month when you menstruate. High levels of ferritin increase your risk of heart disease, so ask your healthcare provider if you need to take iron.

Magnesium. Magnesium plays a central role in thyroid disease. Magnesium is related to the stabilization of the structure of nucleic acids and seems also involved in DNA replication, transcription, and repair. There is a direct link between magnesium and a healthy thyroid and heart related conditions; however, a magnesium deficiency is difficult to test for. You can boost your magnesium intake by eating a well-balanced diet, which includes dark leafy green vegetables, seeds, and nuts, and eliminating caffeine from your diet. Magnesium supplements, such as a pill or magnesium oil, should be taken with caution since they may interact with certain medications. If you are taking any medications, check with your healthcare provider to see if there is a negative interaction.

Molybdenum. Molybdenum is an essential micronutrient. Many studies have found that molybdenum is related to thyroid metabolism. It can interact with thyroid hormone receptors to affect thyroid hormone levels.

Selenium. In the thyroid, selenium is required for the antioxidant function and for the metabolism of thyroid hormones. One study looked at patients that were critically ill and showed that supplementation with selenium normalized thyroid lab results. The literature also suggests that selenium supplementation of patients with autoimmune thyroiditis is associated with a reduction in anti-thyroperoxidase antibody levels, improved thyroid ultrasound features, and improved quality of life. The relevant impact of selenium on inflammatory activity in thyroid-specific autoimmune disease has been shown in several trials demonstrating its possible therapeutic effect in reducing TPOAb in patients with autoimmune thyroiditis. Selenium can exert an influence on immunological responses, cell growth, and viral defense. It is an essential particle in the active site of enzymes such as glutathione peroxidases, deiodinases, and thioredoxin reductases.

In addition, it has a fundamental importance in the synthesis and function of thyroid hormones and protects cells against free radicals and oxidative damage. In fact, selenium demonstrates antioxidant and anti-inflammatory properties that have a relevant impact on immune function, and it has been shown to reduce the inflammatory status in people with Hashimoto's thyroiditis. Adding one or two Brazil nuts or garlic to your diet every day can help to provide you with the needed selenium supplementation. You can get toxic with the use of selenium; therefore, see your doctor or other healthcare provider before starting high doses of selenium as a supplement.

Vitamin B$_2$. Making sure you are getting enough vitamin B$_2$ is necessary in regulating thyroid enzymes and maintaining healthy thyroid function. Eating almonds, eggs in moderation, cashews, salmon, and broccoli help to boost your B$_2$ levels.

Vitamin B$_3$. Vitamin B$_3$ is instrumental in building a strong immune system, and the cause of an underactive thyroid has often been associated with a weak immune system. For a mild vitamin B$_3$ deficiency 50 mg twice a day is recommended.

Vitamin D. Vitamin D is key in keeping your bones strong; however, research suggests that low levels of vitamin D may have an effect on the thyroid working properly, and may influence your immune system. We all need some sun exposure. When skin is exposed to the sun, your body makes vitamin D. However, it only takes a little time in the sun for most people to get the vitamin D they need (and most vitamin D needs should be met with a healthy diet and/or supplements). Visit your healthcare provider to have her vitamin D levels measured to determine your exact dose.

Zinc. Zinc is essential for human health and plays a role in gene expression, cell division and growth, and a variety of enzymes involved in immune and reproductive functioning. Zinc supplementation has also been shown to help with optimal thyroid hormone metabolism. Low levels of zinc in humans can result from a reduced dietary intake and an inadequate absorption of this mineral due to bowel disease or surgery to the bowel. Eating a healthy diet and zinc supplements can be taken to treat a zinc deficiency. However, taking too much zinc can cause toxicity.

Thyroid Hormone Replacement Therapy

When you consider thyroid hormone replacement, it is important to look at how the thyroid hormone is metabolized in the body. The body requires about 50 mg per year of iodine. About 70 percent of the T4 secreted daily is deiodinated to yield T3 and reverse T3 in equal parts. Eighty percent of circulating T3 comes from the peripheral monode-ionization of T4 at the thyrosol ring, which occurs in the liver, kidney, and other tissues. Circulating reverse T3 is made the same way. Thyroid hormone is also metabolized in other pathways. It can be conjugated with glucuronate or sulfate and then excreted in the bile or it can be decarboxylated. Twenty percent to 40 percent of T4 is subsequently eliminated in the stool.

Naltrexone (LDN)

Naltrexone, a non-selective antagonist of opioid receptors, was originally used for drug overdose. In recent years, there have been novel and significant findings on the off-label usage of naltrexone. It is hypothesized that lower than standard doses of naltrexone inhibit cellular proliferation of T and B cells and block Toll-like receptor 4 (protein coding gene), resulting in an analgesic and anti-inflammatory effect. Low-dose naltrexone is a prescription compounded medication that very effectively reduces inflammation. Moreover, LDN can act as an immunomodulator in most autoimmune diseases and malignant tumors as well as alleviate the symptoms of some psychological disorders. LDN is also being used effectively for weight loss as well as prevention and treatment of memory loss.

Mechanisms of Action of LDN

- LDN increases endogenous enkephalins and endorphins, which enhances immune function

- LDN inhibits pro-inflammatory cytokines, which improves the inflammatory reaction

- LDN interacts with nuclear opioid growth factor receptor, which promotes DNA synthesis

- LDN serves as a blockade of opiate-R in GI tract, which heals and repairs the mucosal tissue

Studies have shown that most patients do better, if they need thyroid replacement, to have both T3 and T4 replaced. One study of 89 patients with hypothyroidism that were previously treated with T4 alone was compared to a group of people with low thyroid function that were not treated with T4. The symptoms of the patients already on T4 were not any different from the people who were untreated. In fact, intracellular thyroid hormone receptors have a high affinity for T3. Ninety percent of the thyroid hormone molecules that bind with the receptors are T3 and 10 percent are T4. Other studies have verified that most individuals have less symptoms if they are prescribed both T3 and T4. In another study the lab results were not better, but the patients felt better if they took both T3 and T4.

- LDN regulates Treg and production of IL-10 and TGF-b, which down regulates TH-17

Possible Side Effects
The following are potential short-term side effects of LDN:

- Fatigue
- Hair thinning
- Insomnia (the most common side effect)
- Loss of appetite
- Mild disorientation
- Mood swings
- Nausea
- Vivid dreams

There are also a few potential long-term side effects that may occur with LDN, which include possible liver and kidney toxicity and potential tolerance to the beneficial effects. If you are taking a narcotic, you cannot take low dose naltrexone. Also, if you have hepatitis or liver failure then LDN is contraindicated.

Contact your healthcare provider to discuss the use of LDN, which is a compounded prescription. The dose is ramped up over time, commonly starting with 1.5 mg the first week, 3 mg the second week, and then 4.5 mg thereafter. Many dosage schedules of low-dose naltrexone are currently being used worldwide. It can also be given IV, used topically (transdermally) and intranasally (in the nose).

There are different ways to take thyroid hormone replacement. They are all a prescription. You can take T4 alone, take T3 alone, or take both T4 and T3, which are commonly prescribed as desiccated thyroid, porcine (from a pig). If you have Hashimoto's thyroiditis, some studies in the medical literature suggest that porcine thyroid replacement may not be the best form to take. This problem can be solved by your doctor prescribing non-porcine thyroid hormone, which is compounded. Therefore, it does not have to be made from desiccated thyroid and you would still be able to have a combination of T3 and T4 in one capsule or tablet.

In other words, compounded prescription thyroid medication is customized to your own needs. It is personalized. One size does not fit all patients. Also, you are getting no fillers and the healthcare provider who writes your prescription for compounded thyroid hormone can also add selenium, chromium, zinc, iodine, or other nutrients if needed.

It is crucial that when you start on thyroid medication that you have your thyroid levels re-measured in six weeks. Once you have an optimal dosage schedule then your thyroid level should be re-measured every six months. There are things that can change your dose of thyroid medication, such as weight gain or weight loss. The amount of stress that you have may also affect your thyroid dosage.

Once a diagnosis of Hashimoto's thyroiditis has been confirmed, there are a number of therapies available to treat the condition. With HT, patients should seek to reduce the level of their body's autoimmune response.

- Begin by avoiding all gluten as a lifetime change in your diet. Furthermore, stopping dairy products is beneficial. Also avoid all foods you are allergic to.

- In addition, consider going on a detox diet that pulls out inflammatory foods, which may alleviate thyroid symptoms (see Detoxification section on page 63).

- Next achieving optimal gastrointestinal function may decrease or resolve your symptoms. (See Chapter 11 on Thyroid Hormones and Digestive Health on page 235.) Have your healthcare provider order a gut health test and then follow all of the directions that they suggest to improve your GI health.

- Furthermore, and very importantly, discuss with your healthcare provider starting on low-dose naltrexone (LDN) as a lifetime therapy.

OUTCOME (PROGNOSIS)

While Hashimoto's thyroiditis frequently cannot be cured, it can be well managed. It is imperative for a good outcome that you stop eating gluten, fix the health of your GI tract, and start and stay on low-dose naltrexone (LDN). In addition, by treating HT with thyroid hormones if you have hypothyroidism, normal thyroid hormone levels can be restored, reversing most, if not all, of the signs and symptoms. In addition, by staying away from foods that may increase inflammation in your body, you may avoid worsening your body's immune response. If you are a woman of childbearing age with Hashimoto's, you may have trouble conceiving, so talk to your doctor when planning for a pregnancy.

DISORDERS CAUSED BY OR ASSOCIATED WITH HASHIMOTO'S THYROIDITIS

There are many diseases and conditions that have been associated with Hashimoto's hypothyroidism. Depression has been strongly associated with hypothyroidism, as have heart disease, and memory loss. These disease processes are covered in separate chapters in this book.

Rheumatoid Arthritis

Autoimmune thyroid disease, which is the most common organ-specific autoimmune disorder, is frequently accompanied by other organ and non-organ-specific autoimmune diseases, including rheumatoid arthritis (RA). Although the exact pathogenic mechanisms are still not completely defined, genetics, immune defects, hormones, and environmental factors may play key roles in poly-autoimmunity. Rheumatoid arthritis patients have an increased risk of developing hypothyroidism. This risk was shown to be more common in women and the elderly.

An earlier controlled prospective study found that thyroid dysfunction is almost 3 times greater in patients with RA than in controls without rheumatoid arthritis. Two other studies demonstrated a significant increase in autoimmune thyroiditis patients compared with nontoxic multinodular goiter patients and controls. In addition, a study in The Netherlands also found women with rheumatoid arthritis are three times more likely than the general population of women to develop clinical hypothyroidism, and women with both RA and hypothyroidism are at an elevated risk of developing heart disease. Moreover, a cross-sectional study in Israel comparing 11,782 RA patients and 57,973 controls found that hypothyroidism is more prevalent in rheumatoid patients than in controls. Interestingly, some of the trials suggest that there may be a common genetic link between RA and autoimmune thyroid disease. Family and population studies confirmed the strong genetic influence and inheritability in the development of autoimmune thyroid disease. Autoimmune thyroid disease susceptibility genes can be categorized as either thyroid specific (Tg, TSHR) or immune-modulating (FOXP3, CD25, CD40, CTLA-4, HLA), with HLA-DR3 carrying the highest risk.

The role of genetics in the association of both autoimmune thyroid disease and RA, especially CTLA-4 and PTPN22 polymorphisms is now being discussed in the medical literature. Consequently, if you have rheumatoid arthritis, your healthcare provider should closely monitor you for the development of Hashimoto's hypothyroidism and also Graves' disease.

Chronic Urticaria

Chronic urticaria is a skin disorder defined as the occurrence of daily, or almost daily wheals and itching for at least six weeks. It is a common disease affecting 0.5 percent to 1 percent of the general population. The cause of the disease is still unclear, but there is evidence that autoimmunity and endocrine dysfunction may be involved. The concept of autoimmunity originated from the observation that thyroid disorders and thyroid autoantibodies are more prevalent in individuals with chronic urticaria. Several studies have revealed that there is a significant association between chronic urticaria and thyroid autoimmunity.

CONCLUSION

As you have seen, you can have Hashimoto's thyroiditis, an autoimmune condition where the body is attacking its own thyroid gland, with or without hypothyroidism. The key to treating this disease process is to stop the autoimmune response and then replace thyroid hormone if needed. In the next chapter you will learn about the symptoms, causes, diagnoses, and treatments for hyperthyroidism, when the thyroid makes too much thyroid hormone.

4

Hyperthyroidism

As a general definition, hyperthyroidism usually refers to the over-production of thyroid hormones in the body. However, when you read medical texts, there are two terms that are associated with the over production of thyroid hormones. They are hyperthyroidism and thyrotoxicosis, and while they both refer to the production of too much thyroid hormone in your body, they are two distinctly different conditions.

The term hyperthyroidism refers to disorders that result from long-term overproduction and release of hormones by the thyroid gland. It is a subset of thyrotoxicosis. For individuals with hyperthyroidism, the greater number of symptoms can be very subtle and take several weeks to months to be noticed. This occurs because the slight elevation in thyroid hormones is so small that the patient may not notice or put off going to the doctor. Hyperthyroidism is a long-term condition. The prevalence of hyperthyroidism in the United States is 1.2 percent with overt hyperthyroidism accounting for 0.5 percent of cases. Overt hyperthyroidism happens when the thyroid gland produces too much thyroid hormone and your body goes into overdrive. This condition is also called overactive thyroid. In contrast, subclinical hyperthyroidism accounts for 0.7 percent. Subclinical hyperthyroidism is when TSH levels are low or undetectable but thyroid hormone levels are normal. It commonly is symptomless but may need treatment so that your body does not break down bone structure.

On the other hand, thyrotoxicosis is the clinical manifestation of excess thyroid hormone action at the tissue level due to inappropriately high circulating thyroid hormone concentrations. For example, as will be discussed later, it can be caused by an inflamed or damaged thyroid gland, or by taking or stopping certain drugs. People that have thyrotoxicosis can usually pinpoint the date that their symptoms began and seek medical attention immediately. With a normally functioning thyroid gland, hormones are released into the blood stream over a 30-to-60-day period. In the case of thyrotoxicosis, hormones are released over a shorter period of time, such as a few days or a couple of weeks. This is referred to as a transient hormone excess state. Should thyrotoxicosis occur within an even shorter time frame, this condition is referred to as a thyroid storm or thyroid crisis. It should be considered an emergency and be treated immediately. If left untreated, it can lead to serious illness including death.

The three most common etiologies of hyperthyroidism include:

1. Graves' disease

2. Toxic multinodular goiter

3. Toxic adenoma

Other less common causes of hyperthyroidism:

1. Iodine-induced hyperthyroidism

2. TSH (thyroid stimulating hormone)-secreting pituitary adenomas

3. Conditions associated with high human chorionic gonadotrophin levels: choriocarcinomas and hydatidiform moles in females and germ cell tumors in males

4. Ectopic thyroid in struma ovarii (excess thyroid hormone production from ovarian teratomas)

5. Drug-induced thyroiditis: amiodarone, lithium, tyrosine kinase inhibitors, interferon-alpha, immune checkpoint inhibitor therapy

6. Other thyroiditis: Hashitoxicosis, painless thyroiditis, painful subacute thyroiditis, and suppurative thyroiditis

7. Factitious thyroiditis (due to excess exogenous thyroid hormone: intentional or unintentional use)

8. Infectious thyroiditis

9. Thyroid hormone resistance

As you see, there are several forms hyperthyroidism can take. In order to establish if it is hyperthyroidism, we need to be able to identify the condition and know what the options are. The following section is designed to provide you with such information.

RISK FACTORS

There are risk factors that can increase the possibility of developing hyperthyroidism. The following elements may indicate if an individual is at increased risk.

Age

Hyperthyroidism can occur at any age, but it is more common in people 60 years old or older. On the other hand, Graves' disease usually occurs between the ages of 20 and 40. Graves' disease is an autoimmune form of hyperthyroidism that will be discussed in the next chapter.

Gender

In general, women are more likely to develop hyperthyroidism than men. In regard to Graves' disease, there are eight females for every one male with this specific disease.

Genetics

Statistics strongly indicate that genetics plays a role in a person's predisposition to develop hyperthyroidism. While there is no evidence that only one gene is to blame, it is more likely that the presence of several specific genes increases the incidence of hyperthyroidism. However, in order to turn these genes on, it may require one or more triggers, as listed below, to initiate this condition.

Ethnicity

Statistically, the Japanese appear to be at greater risk for hyperthyroidism than other people. This may be attributed to either genetics or a diet high in iodine rich foods.

CAUSES

When the thyroid is diseased it may produce and release too much thyroid hormone. A number of conditions may be the cause for the overproduction of the thyroid hormone, including:

Emotional and Physical Stress

Recent stress may be a precipitating factor in the development of hyperthyroidism, especially in the class of Graves' disease. The most common precipitating factor is the "actual or threatened" separation from an individual upon whom the patient is emotionally dependent.

Environmental Toxic Exposure

Studies done on lab animals showed that exposure to toxic levels of cadmium and/or mercury increased the risk of developing hyperthyroidism.

Excess Dietary Iodine Supplementation

Thyroid dysfunction due to excess iodine intake is usually mild and transient, but iodine-induced hyperthyroidism can be life-threatening in some individuals. Common sources of iodine are iodized salt, betadine washes, animal milk rich in iodine, drinking water with iodine added, certain seaweeds, iodine-containing dietary supplements, iodine-containing medications, such as amiodarone, radiographic dyes and from a combination of these sources.

A large study looked at the rate of Graves' disease in a population that was required to consume iodized salt. The rate of thyrotoxicosis and Graves' disease was higher throughout the entire study time. The increase in rate included both nodular and diffuse goiters. The conclusion of the study was that iodine supplementation in a group of people that were iodine-sufficient can increase the risk of developing thyrotoxicosis in susceptible people. The median urinary iodine concentration of a population reflects the total iodine intake from all sources and can accurately identify people with excessive iodine intakes. Make sure to talk to your healthcare provider regarding your own situation, and keep track of your iodine levels when your test results come in. Iodine excess may be a problem particularly in people that take iodine without having their iodine levels measured. However, it is important to point out that not having enough iodine can also lead to additional thyroid issues. Iodine levels are best measured by a first morning urine test.

Infections

Special attention is given to patients with hyperthyroidism that have COVID-19 since they may have other complications.

Medications

Some medications, such as amiodarone, lithium, interferon-alpha, IL-2, and GM-CSF (granulocyte-macrophage colony-stimulating factor), can cause an inflammation of the thyroid gland, which in turn can cause an overproduction of thyroid hormones. In addition, taking too much thyroid hormone can lead to hyperthyroidism.

Oxidative Stress

Oxidative stress is also related to hormonal derangement in a reciprocal way. Among the various hormonal influences that operate on the antioxidant balance, thyroid hormones play particularly important roles, since both hyperthyroidism and hypothyroidism have been shown to be associated with oxidative stress. Interestingly, the reverse is also true. Oxidative stress has been shown to be associated with both hyperthyroidism and hypothyroidism. However, the mechanisms by, which oxidative stress is generated in these two clinical conditions are different: increased reactive oxygen species (ROS) production in hyperthyroidism and low availability of antioxidants in hypothyroidism.

Pregnancy and Recent Childbirth

For women going through pregnancy, there are a number of hormonal changes that their bodies experience. This includes increases in progesterone, estrogen, oxytocin, prolactin, and relaxin (a reproductive hormone produced by the ovaries and the placenta to loosen and relax muscles, joints, and ligaments during pregnancy to help the body stretch)—any of these hormones could trigger the development of hyperthyroidism.

Smoking

Smoking has a significant impact on thyroid function interfering with the thyroid's ability to absorb iodine. Oddly enough, in some individuals it can result in an excess amount of thyroid hormone production, and in others, a reduction.

Thyroid Nodules (Toxic Adenoma) (Plummer's Disease)

A benign growth or nodule that has walled itself off from the rest of the gland may cause an enlargement of the thyroid. When this happens the gland may produce an excess amount of the hormone T4, which will then enter into the blood. Toxic adenomas are characterized by a single hyperactive nodule in the thyroid leading to clinical and biochemical thyrotoxicosis. Toxic adenomas are genetic and are related to a somatic mutation in the TSH receptor or Gs alpha subunit. A toxic adenoma is readily recognized on a thyroid scan. Toxic adenomas appear to be more common in countries with a low iodine intake. The possibility of developing thyrotoxicosis in a person with a hot nodule with a diameter of 3 cm or larger is 20 percent within 6 years. This risk is substantially less in smaller nodules. Older individuals with a hot nodule are more likely to become toxic as compared to younger patients. Definitive treatment consists in the administration of 131 iodine, surgical removal of the nodule, or, less commonly used, percutaneous ethanol injection. The risk of malignancy in a toxic nodule is very low. See Chapter 6 on page 119 for further information.

Thyroiditis (Inflamed Thyroid Gland)

The thyroid gland can become inflamed for a variety of reasons. This inflammation can cause the gland to increase in size and to produce excess amounts of thyroid hormone, which will then enter into the bloodstream.

SIGNS AND SYMPTOMS

The following are the most common signs and symptoms of hyperthyroidism and/or thyrotoxicosis. The progression of these individual symptoms, however, may also differ from one individual to another. It is also important to keep in mind that many of these symptoms can be caused by other underlying problems.

Early Symptoms

- Anxiety, nervousness, and irritability

- Brittle fingernails

- Breast enlargement in men (rare)

- Bulging eyes (exophthalmia)

- Constipation

- Diarrhea and/or an increase in bowel movements

- Difficulty in managing diabetes

- Elevated heart rate (tachycardia) and/or chest pain

- Erectile dysfunction or reduced sexual urges

- Eyelid retraction, puffy eyelids, reddening around the eyes, pressure on the eyes, and irritation of the eyes as well as double vision (Graves' thyroid eye disease)

- Goiter (enlargement of the thyroid gland)

- Heart palpitations (sensation heart is pounding)

- Heat or cold intolerance

- Muscle weakness

- Personality or psychological changes

- Perspiring profusely (diaphoresis)

- Separation of nail from the nail bed (onycholysis)

- Shortness of breath

- Skin changes

- Slight trembling of the hands or fingers

- Weight change (weight loss or gain)

Late Symptoms

- Decreased ability to hear

- Hoarseness

- Lumpy thickening and reddening of the skin, usually on the shins or tops of the feet (Graves' dermopathy)

- Menstrual disorders

- Puffy face, hands, and feet

- Slow speech

- Thinning eyebrow hair

Symptoms can also be grouped under classifications concerning the area of the body they occur in:

General

- Fatigue

- Heat intolerance

- Increased appetite

- Increased sweating from cutaneous blood flow increase

- Onycholysis (separation of nails from nail beds)

- Pretibial myxedema (a skin condition that causes plaques of thick, scaly skin and swelling of your lower legs)

- Weakness

- Weight loss

Eyes

- Graves' ophthalmopathy (also called Graves' eye disease)

- Lid lag (when looking down, sclera visible above cornea)

- Lid retraction (when looking straight, sclera visible above the cornea)

Goiter

- Diffuse, smooth, non-tender goiter

- The audible bruit can be heard at the superior poles of the thyroid gland

Cardiovascular

- Abnormal heart rhythms

- An irregular pulse from atrial fibrillation

- Chest pain

- Heart failure (occurs much more commonly in elderly patients)

- Hypertension (high blood pressure)

- Palpitations (heart racing, pounding, missing a beat, having an extra beat)

- Tachycardia (heart racing, which can be masked by people taking beta-blockers)

- Widened pulse pressure because systolic pressure increases and diastolic pressure decreases

Musculoskeletal

- Fine tremors of the outstretched fingers. Face, tongue, and head can also be involved. Tremors respond well to treatment with beta-blockers.

- Myopathy (disease of the muscle) affects proximal muscles. Serum creatine kinase (CK) levels can be normal.

- Osteoporosis (bone loss)

Neuropsychiatric system

- Anxiety
- Depression
- Drug-induced
- Emotional instability

- Hyperreflexia (overactive bodily reflexes)
- Insomnia
- Restlessness
- Tremulousness

Most commonly, younger individuals tend to show symptoms of sympathetic activation—that is, the fight or flight response—which brings on anxiety, hyperactivity, and tremors. With patients over 60, the symptoms may more frequently involve cardiovascular related issues, which need to be carefully monitored.

TESTING

If you are experiencing any of the symptoms associated with hyperthyroidism, there are a number of tests available to determine whether you have hyperthyroidism or thyrotoxicosis.

Physical Examination

Normally, a physician can see some of the more pronounced signs, such goiters, thyroid enlargement, or signs of tremors, which can indicate hyperthyroidism.

Blood Tests

In a standard blood test, there is usually an increase in the level of thyroid hormones (T3 and T4) in individuals that have overt hyperthyroidism. There is also a compensatory decrease in the level of the thyroid-stimulating hormone (TSH) since the thyroid is now being stimulated by an antibody, TSH production would naturally drop. In another specialized blood test, the level of the thyroid peroxidase antibody (TPO) is measured. This may indicate that there is an autoimmune disorder present. However, since 5 percent to 10 percent of healthy individuals test positive for TPO, the results of this antibody test may not be conclusive. If the tests all come back within a normal range, these blood tests can at least rule out hyperthyroidism.

Fine Needle Aspiration (FNA)

If a node is found, a fine needle aspiration is done. The skin above the node is numbed, and a thin needle is inserted into the node to remove cells and fluid for review. These samples are then sent to a laboratory where a pathologist examines them under a microscope to determine the exact nature of the cells. The pathologist writes up a report on the findings and sends back the report to the ordering physician.

While the FNA is designed to determine if the cells are benign or cancerous, up to 30 percent of the FNA biopsies may be inconclusive. When this happens a blood test may be able to provide an answer. However, should it not, traditionally, surgery is the next step to determine if the node is benign or cancerous. Recently, however, a new personalized genetic test has been developed to provide an answer based on the initial FNA biopsy, which can help prevent unnecessary surgeries. (See "Personalized Genetic Tests" below.)

Personalized Genetic Tests

Beyond just testing for inherited thyroid cancer-prone genes, there are new personalized genetic tests available, which may be able to rule out whether the cells taken from a FNA procedure are benign or malignant. Additionally, the tests may also be able to determine how aggressive a cancerous thyroid cell may be. These tests are based upon molecular identification. The results of such tests can enable a surgeon to determine how extensive a surgery is needed or if one is required at all. (See Chapter 18 on page 297 for more on thyroid cancer.)

Ultrasound of the Thyroid

Ultrasound imaging is used to determine the size and vascularity of the thyroid gland and the location, size, number, and characteristics of thyroid nodules.

Radioactive Iodine Uptake (RAIU)

A radioactive iodine uptake test (RAIU) is designed to measure the amount of iodine your thyroid absorbs and determine whether all or only part of the thyroid is overactive. The amount of radioactive tracer your thyroid absorbs determines if your thyroid function is normal or abnormal. A high uptake of iodine tracer may mean you have hyperthyroidism.

Scan of the Area Around Your Eyes

If the patient is showing either irritation around the eye and eye socket or there is a bulging of the eyes, a number of scans can be ordered. Ultrasound, magnetic resonance imaging (MRI) or computed tomography (CT) scan may be performed to determine the extent of impact the irritation has caused.

Thyroid Scan

A radioactive iodine tracer is injected into the vein in the arm or hand. You then lie on a table with a scanner that produces an image of your thyroid on a computer screen. The image can show whether parts of the thyroid gland are absorbing too much or too little of the radioactive iodine. This test may be given as part of a radioactive iodine uptake test. In that case, orally administered radioactive iodine is normally used to image the thyroid gland.

Thyroid Scintigraphy with either Radioactive Iodine or Tc-pertechnetate

Thyroid scintigraphy is a medical procedure that allows the function of the thyroid gland to be assessed. Scintigraphy consists of administering either radioiodine or ^{99m}Tc-pertechnetate is useful to characterize different forms of hyperthyroidism and provides information for planning radioiodine therapy.

Based upon the patient's family history, risk factors, symptoms, and test results, the doctor will determine if the problem is hyperthyroidism.

TREATMENT

The treatment of choice for hyperthyroidism is governed by many factors. It depends on age, goiter size and association with nodular disease, existence of Graves' eye disease, standard of care in the area in, which one lives, the personal preference of the treating physician, any other disease processes one may have, and of course the patient's choice. Treatment of thyroid storm is a medical emergency and must be treated immediately. The goal of these treatments is to correct the overproduction of thyroid hormone. The following is a summary of common treatments for hyperthyroidism and thyrotoxicosis. Also see the chapters on Graves' disease and thyroid disorders caused by, or associated with, hyperthyroidism and thyrotoxicosis.

Anti-thyroid Medication

One of the first options in the treatment of hyperthyroidism is anti-thyroid medications. Anti-thyroid drugs are designed to interfere with the thyroid gland's ability to produce hormones thereby decreasing hormone production. Unlike other treatments, once they are discontinued, they allow the thyroid to function as usual. Side effects many vary with each drug. These may include nausea, vomiting, heartburn, headache, rash, joint pain, loss of taste, liver failure, or a decrease in disease-fighting white blood cells. Pregnant women should always check with their doctor regarding when they can start on such medications. These drugs can usually be discontinued once a stable normal thyroid balance has been achieved with other therapies. However, recurrence of hyperthyroidism after a 12 to 18 month course of antithyroid drugs occurs in approximately 50 percent of patients. Being younger than 40 years, having free T4 concentrations that are 40 pmol/L or higher, having TSH-binding inhibitory immunoglobulins that are higher than 6 U/L, and having a goiter size that is equivalent to or larger than WHO grade 2 before the start of treatment with antithyroid drugs increase risk of recurrence. Long-term treatment with antithyroid drugs (for example, 5 to 10 years of treatment) is feasible and associated with fewer recurrences (15 percent) than short-term treatment (for example, 12-18 months of treatment).

Let's take a closer look at some of the other medications.

Beta blockers (B-Adrenergic Antagonist Drugs). Beta blockers were originally designed to reduce blood pressure by blocking the effects of epinephrine, also called adrenaline. It does this by slowing down the number of heartbeats per minute as well as opening up blocked vessels. This, in turn, reduces tachycardia, palpitations, tremor, and anxiety. The effects of beta blockers are fast, so it is important for use early on in the treatment of thyrotoxicosis. These drugs do not affect thyroid function, release, or synthesis. Beta blockers should not be used if you have asthma, emphysema, congestive heart failure, bradycardia (slow heartbeat), hypotension (low blood pressure), COPD (chronic obstructive pulmonary disease), or Raynaud's phenomenon.

Iodine and iodine-containing compounds. Pharmacologic doses of iodine as Lugol's solution or saturated solution of potassium iodide (SSKI) work by the following mechanisms:

- Decrease iodine transport into the thyroid

- Inhibit iodine organification in the thyroid gland, thereby diminishing thyroid hormone biosynthesis, a phenomenon called Wolff-Chaikoff effect

- Decrease the vascularity of the thyroid in Graves' disease

The effects are transient, lasting only a few days to weeks. Thyrotoxicosis may return and even worsen. Consequently, iodine therapy is used only short term in preparation for surgery after a normal state has been achieved and maintained with the use of thionamides. Iodine is also used to treat thyroid storm since it can inhibit thyroid hormone immediately.

Oral cholecystographic agents. Oral cholecystographic agents (iodine containing radiocontrast agents), such as iopanoic acid and sodium ipodate, produce a rapid fall in thyroid hormones. They act by inhibition of the peripheral conversion of T4 to T3 and by prevention of thyroid hormone secretion because of the inorganic iodine that is released from the drug. Both iopanoic acid and sodium ipodate because of their rapid onset of action are very effective treatments for thyrotoxicosis. They are not effective for long-term treatment because of the escape of thyroid hormone synthesis from the blocking action of iodine. Furthermore, iopanoic acid and sodium ipodate provide a load of iodine to the thyroid, which makes the using of radioactive iodine not feasible for weeks. Therefore, these drugs are best used for emergency situations for a rapid decrease in thyroid hormone production or prior to surgery.

Perchlorate. Perchlorate works by inhibiting the transport of iodine into the thyroid. Possible side effects include stomach irritation and aplastic anemia. These side effects are somewhat common; therefore, it stops the use of perchlorate as treatment for hyperthyroidism/thyrotoxicosis long-term.

Used in conjunction with thionamides, perchlorate has been used successfully for depleting the thyroidal iodine overload in amiodarone-induced hyperthyroidism.

Thionamides. There are three thionamides drugs, methimazole (MMI), carbimazole, and propylthiouracil (PTU), which are effective in their treatment of hyperthyroidism. Thionamides do not block the release of preformed thyroid hormone. They inhibit thyroid peroxidase, blocking the making of T3 and T4. Consequently, it takes 1 to 6 weeks for the thyroid hormones that are already stored and the iodine that is stored to be depleted and the patient to have total relief of symptoms and normalization of thyroid studies. Large goiters with large deposits of thyroid hormone may show a delayed response to thionamides. Thionamides represent the treatment of choice in pregnant women, during lactation, in children and adolescents and in preparation for radioiodine therapy or thyroidectomy (removal of the thyroid gland).

The main problem with the use of thionamides is that there is a high relapse rate of thyrotoxicosis when the medications are stopped. Recurrence rate is 50 to 80 percent depending on the length of follow-up. Most relapses occur within 3 to 6 months, but it can occur much later. Remission rates have decreased over the last decade, perhaps due to an increased iodine supply in the diet of the average American. Relapse to hyperthyroidism after treatment suggests that another form of treatment may be necessary such as ablative therapy. Some people become hypothyroid after therapy.

Mild side effects have been reported in 1 to 15 percent of patients that take thionamides.

- Hives (urticaria)
- Itching (pruritus)
- Joint pain (arthralgias)
- Slightly elevated liver enzymes
- Skin rash

Severe side effects of thioamides are rare and require prompt discontinuation of the medication.

- Cholestatic necrotic hepatitis
- Decrease of white blood cells (agranulocytosis)
- Inflammation of blood vessels (vasculitis)
- Lupus-like syndrome
- Toxic hepatitis

Thionamides can serve as a long-term therapy or as a bridge to I-131 ablation or thyroidectomy (thyroid surgery), with the goal of normalizing thyroid function and preventing exacerbation of hyperthyroidism after I-131 ablation or avoiding surgical risks associated with uncontrolled hyperthyroidism. Because Graves' disease (see the next chapter for more information) remits in up to 30 percent of patients treated with thionamides, these medications can be used as the initial treatment, with ablation or thyroidectomy performed if remission does not occur. Once medical therapy is discontinued, relapse occurs in 30 percent to 70 percent of people, mostly within the first year. After discontinuation, thyroid function should be monitored by your healthcare provider on a regular basis. Contact your physician if symptoms recur.

Radioactive Iodine Therapy

As discussed earlier, in order to function, the thyroid gland needs to absorb iodine on a daily basis. With this therapy, a radioactive form of iodine is orally taken by the patient. As the reactive iodine is absorbed, the low-level radiation is enough to destroy the overactive thyroid cells causing the thyroid to shrink and to produce less hormones.

Because this treatment involves destroying thyroid cells, it will likely influence the amount of thyroid hormones produced in the future. For that reason, a patient's thyroid hormone levels must be checked regularly, and that individual may require thyroid medication to make up for a drop in thyroid hormone production.

This treatment may not be effective in patients with large goiters; consequently, several treatments may be needed. If you have a large goiter, then surgery may be the therapy of choice. In the elderly, radioactive iodine is usually the treatment of choice. In women that are of childbearing age, they should delay pregnancy for 6 to 12 months after receiving radioactive iodine.

Surgery

Another possible treatment for hyperthyroidism is surgery. The goal of surgery is to decrease the excessive secretion of thyroid hormone and to prevent a relapse of thyrotoxicosis. For a long time, partial thyroidectomy was recommended. Recently, total thyroidectomy (the entire thyroid gland is removed) is more commonly performed. There is a higher rate of hypothyroidism associated with this procedure, but a lower rate of recurrence of hyperthyroidism.

Commonly your doctor will have you treated with thioamide, an anti-thyroid medication, to restore and maintain a normal thyroid state in preparation for surgery. The thionamides act by multiple mechanisms. The major action is to prevent hormone synthesis by inhibiting the thyroid peroxidase-catalyzed reactions and blocking iodine organification. In addition, they block coupling of the iodotyrosines. Adverse effects of thionamides include common, minor side effects (for example, a rash) and rare but serious adverse effects, such as agranulocytosis (deficiency of granulocytes, which increases your risk of developing an infection) and hepatotoxicity (liver toxicity). Surgeons may use inorganic iodine 10 days before surgery to induce the involution of the thyroid gland and decrease the vascularity, which makes the surgery easier.

Surgery is the best choice for individuals that have a larger goiter, or if cancer cannot be ruled out, if cancer is present, and if multiple cold nodules are not expected to respond with shrinkage to radioactive iodine.

Some of the possible side effects of surgery include infection, bleeding, thyroid storm, injury to the recurrent laryngeal nerve, hypoparathyroidism, hypothyroidism, and hypocalcemia (low calcium level). With the partial or whole removal of your thyroid gland, levels of thyroid hormones must be carefully monitored.

PERSOANLIZED MEDICINE THERAPIES FOR HYPERTHYRODISM AND THYROTOXICOSIS

There are natural therapies for hyperthyroidism that have been shown to be clinically effective for *mild* disease. For moderate or severe hyperthyroidism and for any forms of thyrotoxicosis, natural therapies alone are not recommended. These may commonly, however, be used in conjunction with standard medical treatment. Before starting any of these therapies, each natural option should be discussed with your healthcare provider.

Acupuncture

Acupuncture, the use of small needles strategically placed in the skin, has been used as a treatment in China for thousands of years. Studies in China have shown it to be effective in treating hyperthyroidism.

Cold packs

By placing ice packs over the thyroid gland, found at the base of your neck, three times a day, you can reduce swelling. (See Figure 1.2 on page 10.) The cold will also help slow down the function of the thyroid gland.

Diet

In treating your hyperthyroidism, it is important to learn how to get as much nutrition as possible from your food and to learn to make good food choices.

Eat Foods That Are Good For You

Whole fruits, vegetables, and nuts head the list. In addition, a high protein diet has been shown to be effective against mild hyperthyroidism.

These foods contain goitrogens, a naturally occurring chemical, which has been shown to prevent or make it more difficult to utilize iodine. In so doing, they block thyroid synthesis. These goitrogenic foods include:

- Almonds
- Broccoli
- Brussels sprouts
- Cabbage
- Cassava root
- Cauliflower
- Kohlrabi (a vegetable)
- Millet
- Mustard
- Peaches
- Peanuts
- Pine nuts
- Rapeseeds
- Rutabagas
- Soybeans
- Sweet potatoes
- Turnips

However, it is important to understand these foods cannot be reliably used in place of medications in the treatment of hyperthyroidism since their goitrogen content is low. Furthermore, cooking inactivates the goitrogens. Likewise, no substantial documentation is available to show that dietary goitrogens interfere with thyroid function if the patient has adequate levels of iodine.

Studies have shown, moreover, that individuals with hyperthyroidism should eat foods that contain flavonoids since they decrease serum T4 and inhibit both the conversion of T4 to T3 and 5'deiodinase activity. Foods such as fruits and vegetables of yellow, orange, red, and purple color, such as blueberries, purple grapes, and cherries, contain flavonoids.

Limiting Your Food Choices

In addition to eating the right foods, you can minimize your hyperthyroid symptoms by avoiding certain foods and drinks.

Avoid caffeine. Caffeine can increase the severity of many symptoms of hyperthyroidism, such as rapid heart rate, anxiety, and tremors. By eliminating products such as soda, coffee, tea, and chocolate from your diet, you can control some of these persistent issues.

Avoid foods that contain iodine. Foods that are high in iodine, such as seaweeds, iodized salt, fish from the sea, and shellfish, should be avoided.

Avoid foods that you are allergic to. While it may be easy to identify foods and avoid the foods you are allergic to, some people have hidden food allergies that they may not be aware of. (See Chapter 11 on page 235.) Many of these food allergies can aggravate symptoms of hyperthyroidism. Make sure you are aware of all the foods you may have allergies to.

Avoid processed foods. Cut down or stop consuming foods that are heavily processed, salted, and/or sugared. Find a healthful diet that you can stick to.

Nutritional Supplements

Nutritional supplements may be helpful in the treatment of mild hyperthyroidism. Free radical injury occurs when the body is exposed to excess thyroid hormone. Furthermore, low antioxidant status has been found in patients with excess thyroid production. In fact, the degree of cell damage in hyperthyroidism has been shown to be directly correlated with the amount of oxidative stress that is present. Taking antioxidants such as vitamins A, C, and E have been shown to be helpful alone or in conjunction with medications.

Calcium Citrate. Calcium metabolism may be changed in hyperthyroidism where patients with hyperthyroidism have an increased risk of developing osteoporosis. Supplementing with calcium may be beneficial.

Coenzyme Q-10. Similar to a vitamin, this substance is a cofactor in the electron-transport chain, which is the energy producing cycle in the body. Q-10 levels have been shown to be low in adults and children with hyperthyroidism. Studies have also shown that coenzyme Q-10 levels may return to normal after treatment of hyperthyroidism with conventional therapies. It may be helpful to supplement Q-10 in people with hyperthyroidism that have cardiac disease and also in individuals with longstanding uncorrected hyperthyroidism.

L-carnitine. This amino acid is used for the transport of long-chain fatty acids into the mitochondria. L-carnitine is an antagonist of thyroid hormone in peripheral tissues by inhibiting thyroid hormone entry into the nucleus of the cells. One study conducted over 6 months used carnitine in patients with hyperthyroidism. Patients taking L-carnitine improved their symptoms and liver profiles, but the patients that did not take L-carnitine were worse. The form of L-carnitine used should be L-carnitine alone or the acetic or propionic acid form and not the D-form. If you have compromised kidney function, you may not be able to take L-carnitine or the dose may need to be decreased, therefore contact your physician before taking L-carnitine. You cannot take L-carnitine if you have an elevated TMAO level. Have your doctor measure your TMAO level, which is a fasting blood study, before starting this nutrient.

Selenium. Subclinical (undetected) hyperthyroidism may be due to low selenium intake. In fact, selenium deficiency alters the conversion of T4 to T3 in peripheral tissues such as the kidney and the liver. One study found men fed low selenium diets had their serum T3 levels increase. A medical trial showed that subjects with autoimmune thyroiditis were given 200 micrograms of selenium for 3 months and their antibodies decreased or resolved. Selenium is one of the supplements that should be considered as a therapy for mild hyperthyroidism in people that are not high in selenium or selenium toxic.

Vitamin A. Given in large doses, this antioxidant has an inhibitory effect on the thyroid gland. Vitamin A supplementation has been shown to decrease the symptoms of hyperthyroidism. The exact mechanism by, which vitamin A works is unknown. If you smoke, then do not consider this therapy, since large doses of vitamin A in smokers may be linked to an increased risk of developing lung cancer.

Vitamin C (Ascorbic acid). Animal studies have shown that thyroid hormone in excess can reduce ascorbic acid levels in the blood, liver, adrenal glands, thymus, and kidney. Studies in human trials in patients with hyperthyroidism have also shown an increase in excretion of ascorbic acid. Furthermore, trials have shown that the medications thiourea and thiouracil also lower ascorbic acid levels. Consequently, supplementation with vitamin C is suggested in patients with hyperthyroidism. Supplementation does not affect the course of the disease, but it may decrease the symptoms and metabolic effects.

Vitamin E. This vitamin may be protective against the oxidative damage caused by hyperthyroidism. In an animal study, animals with hyperthyroidism were given vitamin E, which helped to prevent the lipid peroxidation that is associated with hyperthyroidism. Human studies have shown that individuals with hyperthyroidism have low vitamin E levels. Consequently, supplementation with vitamin E is suggested.

Zinc. Red blood cell zinc levels are lower in patients with hyperthyroidism since zinc needs are increased because of greater urinary zinc excretion in this disease process. Therapy with anti-thyroid medications has been shown to normalize RBC zinc levels 2 months after free T3 and free T4 have been normalized.

Herbs

There are several botanical supplements that may be helpful in some patients with mild hyperthyroidism. It is always advisable to work with a trained professional when using herbal supplementation.

Bugleweed. The German Commission E, Germany's equivalent to the FDA, recognizes the use of bugleweed for mild hyperthyroid conditions associated with the dysfunction of the nervous system based on pharmacologic studies. However, they also stated that in rare situations high dosages have resulted in thyroid enlargement and sudden discontinuation has increased disease symptoms.

Club moss. This herb has been studied for hyperthyroidism like bugleweed. Animal studies using club moss have shown its ability to block TSH activity at the receptor level, block the release of TSH from the thyroid, and suppress the iodine pump. It can also inhibit the peripheral T4 deiodination and conversion to T3.

Emblica officinalis. Animal studies using Emblica officinalis are promising. It was shown to reduce T3 and T4 concentrations by a significant amount. Human trials need to be done.

Flavonoids. There are also botanical medicines that contain flavonoids, such as hawthorne berry, astragalus, ginkgo biloba, licorice, and chamomile, which may be helpful for mild hyperthyroidism.

Ginger. It has been found that ginger has a positive effect on thyroid function. Ginger contains magnesium, which has been proven to be a key factor in controlling thyroid disease. Since it aids in regulating inflammation, it is also considered to protect against thyroid conditions that are caused by inflammation. Ginger can be used in various ways. Fresh ginger root can be added when cooking or baking in the diced or powder form. In pill form, start with one capsule, twice a day.

Lemon balm. This herb has calming effects on the nervous system and has been used since ancient times for this issue. Lab studies have confirmed lemon balm's ability to block TSH receptors and inhibit both binding of bovine TSH to human thyroid tissue, and binding of autoantibodies in Graves' disease. Lemon balm has been used extensively in individuals with mild hyperthyroidism.

Motherwort. This is used traditionally to treat anxiety, depression, heart palpitations, and tachycardia (heart racing). Therefore, it may be good for relief of symptoms of mild hyperthyroidism. It can be used with bugleweed. The German Commission E supports the use of motherwort for the treatment of cardiac disorders associated with anxiety and for the symptomatic relief of mild hyperthyroidism.

Turmeric. Turmeric is an herb that has been used for thousands of years. Like ginger, it can be beneficial in treating inflammation. It has anti-inflammatory properties, which help to treat thyroid dysfunctions such as Graves' disease and other inflammatory forms of hyperthyroidism. You can add turmeric when cooking or it can be taken in capsule form. Follow dosage directions on the package.

OUTCOME (PROGNOSIS)

Once the source of the hyperthyroidism has been identified and eliminated, the overproduction of thyroid hormones should stop. However, as a result of a number of treatments, there can now be a permanent under-production of thyroid hormones, which can lead to hypothyroidism. (See page 25.) When this happens, patients are put on thyroid hormone for the remainder of their lives in order to normalize their thyroid hormone levels. Once done, all the symptoms and signs of hypothyroidism should be reversed.

CONCLUSION

As you have seen in this chapter, hyperthyroidism is more common than you may have realized. It can go undetected for years, appearing as any number of health issues. While it may not be immediately recognized for what it is, by understanding what causes it and what to look for, you can be your own best advocate. As you have seen in this chapter, there are many therapies, both conventional and natural, that have been found to be effective for hyperthyroidism.

While this chapter has provided you with a general overview of hyperthyroidism, there are more specific types of hyperthyroidism. We will examine these other forms in the next couple of chapters. The next chapter (Chapter 5) will examine Graves' disease. Chapter 6 will take a closer look at the other categories of hyperthyroidism/thyrotoxicosis.

5

Graves' Disease

As you will see in the next chapter, there are various causes and treatments related to hyperthyroidism and thyrotoxicosis. Graves' disease is the most common cause of hyperthyroidism. It is an autoimmune disease caused by the production of TSH receptor antibodies that stimulate thyroid gland growth and thyroid hormone release. Individuals with this disease will have abnormally increased T4 and T3 levels and a decrease in TSH.

A positive TSH-receptor IgG immunoglobulin test confirms the diagnosis in, which the level is abnormally high in people with hyperthyroidism due to Graves' disease. Immunoglobulin G (IgG) against the TSH-receptor leads to increased thyroid function and growth. Individuals will often present with symptoms of hyperthyroidism and diffuse goiter. TSH-receptor antibodies can also activate orbital (within the eye) fibroblasts leading to fibroblast proliferation, and differentiation to adipocytes (a cell that stores fat). As a result, there is elevated production of hyaluronic acid and glycosaminoglycan (GAG), leading to an increased volume of intraorbital fat and muscle tissue. It causes exophthalmos (where the eyeball protrudes from the eye socket, making it appear to bulge), lid retraction, and diplopia (double vision) due to ocular motility problems. Up to 50 percent of patients with Graves' disease develop thyroid eye disease (TED). Pretibial myxedema (a skin condition that causes plaques of thick, scaly skin and swelling of your lower legs) is another finding in Graves' disease. It is due to the stimulation of dermal fibroblasts that leads to depositions of GAGs in the connective tissue.

Graves' disease, as just discussed, is the most common form of hyperthyroidism. It is also known as diffuse toxic goiter and Flajani-Basedow Graves' disease. It represents 85 percent of all hyperthyroid cases. It is considered an autoimmune disease because of the way in, which the body's immune system works against itself.

As we learned in Chapter 1, the pituitary gland produces thyroid stimulating hormone (TSH). TSH in turn triggers the thyroid gland into producing enough T3 and T4 hormones that the body requires. For any number of reasons, in this autoimmune process, the body's immune system produces thyrotropin receptor antibody (TRAb) that acts in the same way TSH does, simulating the thyroid tissue to overproduce T3 and T4. In some cases, the symptoms may be mild, while in other cases, the symptoms can be serious. Normally in Graves' disease, the entire thyroid gland becomes enlarged.

Graves' disease also occurs in 3 to 5 percent of people who have myasthenia gravis, a degenerative muscular disease.

RISK FACTORS

The flare-up of antibodies that are at the root cause of Graves' disease can be initiated by any number of reasons. The following factors may indicate if an individual is at a higher risk.

Age

The signs of Graves' disease usually present between the ages of 20 and 40.

Gender

For every one male patient with Graves' disease there are eight females. However, the ratio of patients that develop eye complications is equal in both men and women. Women with normal hormone levels of the estrogen, but with an increased sensitivity to the estrogen, have a higher prevalence of antibodies that may affect the thyroid.

Genetics

Statistics strongly indicate that genetics plays a role in a person's predisposition to develop Graves' disease. While there is no evidence that only one gene is to blame, it is more likely that the presence of several specific genes increases the incidence of Graves' disease. Research has shown that Graves' disease is passed on from one generation to another and shows up in identical twins. However, it may require one or more triggers, as listed below, to initiate this condition.

Left-Handedness

Oddly enough, a study done by Wood and Cooper showed a statistically significant trend for left-handed people to be affected by Graves' disease.

CAUSES

Although Graves' disease has been studied for years, its causes remain unclear. There are, however, some conditions that are thought to be likely triggers.

Emotional and Physical Stress

Recent stress may be a precipitating factor in the development of Graves' disease. The most common precipitating factor is the actual or threatened separation from an individual upon whom the patient is emotionally dependent. Furthermore, studies now support the idea that Graves' disease often follows an emotional shock.

Existing Autoimmune Diseases

Graves' disease is caused by a breakdown in the body's disease-fighting immune system. For those people with preexisting immune system disorders, such as type 1 diabetes or rheumatoid arthritis, studies have shown that there is an increased risk of developing Graves' disease.

Infections

Viral and bacterial infections have been reported in a large percentage of patients with Graves' disease. Studies indicate that a number of these pathogens can trigger the body's immune system to create antibodies; and it is in the body's natural response that a specific antibody may attach itself to the thyroid cells to overproduce hormones.

Studies have reported an increase in the frequency of anti-influenza B virus antibodies found in patients with thyrotoxicosis. A large prevalence of circulating antibodies against the bacteria *Yersinia enterocolitica*, strain 0:3 have been seen in patients with Graves' disease. Also, *Yersinia* antibodies have been found to interact with thyroid structures. Low-affinity binding sites for TSH have been found in other bacteria—*Leishmania* and *Mycoplasma*. Retroviral sequences or proteins have also been found in the thyroid gland of patients with Graves' disease. This may be due to a secondary infection.

Special attention is given to patients with Graves' disease that have COVID-19 since they may have other complications.

Oxidative Stress

Oxidative stress is involved in the pathogenesis of Graves' hyperthyroidism and Graves' orbitopathy (eye disease) due to the increased reactive oxygen species (ROS) production that commonly occurs in all forms of hyperthyroidism. The elevation in ROS is due to an imbalance of the cell oxidation-reduction, or redox reaction, which is a reaction that involves the transfer of electrons between chemical states. An increase in ROS production is commonly associated with thyroid hyperfunction (over-production).

Pregnancy and Recent Childbirth

For women going through pregnancy, there are a number of hormonal changes that their bodies experience. This includes increases in progesterone, estrogen, oxytocin, prolactin, and relaxin (a reproductive hormone produced by the ovaries and the placenta to loosen and relax muscles, joints, and ligaments during pregnancy to help the body stretch). Any one of these or a combination of these hormones could trigger the development of Graves' disease.

Smoking

Studies showed a relatively small correlation between smoking and Graves' thyroid eye disease. There also appears to be an increase in symptoms when smoking is combined with drugs designed to stop the overproduction of thyroid hormones.

SIGNS AND SYMPTOMS

The following are the common signs and symptoms of Graves' disease. The progression of these, however, may also differ from one individual to another. It is also important to keep in mind that many of these symptoms can be caused by other underlying problems.

- Anxiety, nervousness, and irritability
- Breast enlargement in men (rare)
- Bulging eyes (exophthalmia)
- Chest pains and/or rapid or irregular heartbeat (palpitations)

- Difficulty in managing diabetes

- Erectile dysfunction or reduced sexual urges

- Eyelid retraction, puffy eyelids, reddening around the eyes, pressure on the eyes, and irritation of the eyes as well as double vision (Graves' thyroid eye disease)

- Goiter (enlargement of the thyroid gland)

- Heat intolerance

- Increase in bowel movements and/or diarrhea

- Lumpy thickening and reddening of the skin, usually on the shins or tops of the feet (Graves' dermopathy)

- Personality or psychological changes

- Perspiring profusely (diaphoresis)

- Shortness of breath

- Slight trembling of the hands or fingers

- Thinning hair

- Weight change (weight loss or gain)

Symptoms can also be grouped under classifications concerning the area of the body they occur in:

General

- Fatigue

- Heat intolerance

- Increased appetite

- Increased sweating from cutaneous blood flow increase

- Onycholysis (separation of nails from nail beds)

- Pretibial myxedema (a skin condition that causes plaques of thick, scaly skin and swelling of your lower legs)

- Weakness

- Weight loss

Eyes

- Graves' ophthalmopathy (also called Graves' eye disease)

- Lid lag (when looking down, sclera visible above cornea)

- Lid retraction (when looking straight, sclera visible above the cornea)

Goiter

- Diffuse, smooth, non-tender goiter

- The audible bruit can be heard at the superior poles of the thyroid gland

Cardiovascular

- Abnormal heart rhythms

- An irregular pulse from atrial fibrillation

- Chest pain

- Heart failure (occurs most commonly in elderly patients)

- Hypertension (high blood pressure)

- Palpitations (heart racing, pounding, missing a beat, having an extra beat)

- Tachycardia (heart racing, which can be masked by people taking beta-blockers)

- Widened pulse pressure because systolic pressure increases and diastolic pressure decreases

Musculoskeletal

- Fine tremors of the outstretched fingers. Face, tongue, and head can also be involved. Tremors respond well to treatment with beta-blockers.

- Myopathy (disease of the muscle) affects proximal muscles. Serum creatine kinase (CK) levels can be normal.

- Osteoporosis (bone loss)

Neuropsychiatric system

- Anxiety

- Depression

- Drug-induced

- Emotional instability

- Hyperreflexia (overactive bodily reflexes)

- Insomnia

- Restlessness

- Tremulousness

Most commonly, younger patients tend to show symptoms of sympathetic activation—that is, the fight or flight response—which brings on anxiety, hyperactivity, and tremors. With people over 60, the symptoms may more frequently involve cardiovascular related issues, which need to be carefully monitored. If you think you have the onset of Graves' disease, review the tests listed below that are available to you, to evaluate your condition, and see your healthcare provider.

TESTING

There are several tests available to determine whether you have Graves' disease or another potential form of hyperthyroidism.

Physical Examination

Normally, a physician can see some of the more pronounced signs, such as irritated or bulging eyes, thyroid enlargement, or signs of tremors, which can indicate Graves' disease.

Blood Tests

Thyroid Peroxidase Antibody (TPO)

In a standard blood test, there would be an increase in the level of thyroid hormones (T3 and T4) as would be expected with hyperthyroidism, and there would be a decrease in the level of the thyroid-stimulating hormone (TSH). Because the thyroid is now being stimulated by an antibody, TSH production would naturally drop. In another specialized blood test, the level of the thyroid peroxidase antibody (TPO) is measured. This may indicate that there is an autoimmune disorder present. However, since 5 percent to 10 percent of healthy individuals test positive for TPO, the results of this antibody test may not be conclusive. If the tests all come back within a normal range, these blood tests can at least rule out Graves' disease.

Thyrotropin Receptor Antibody Test (TRAb)

The thyrotropin receptor antibody (TRAb) test is a blood test that is used to diagnose Graves' disease. The antibodies it tests for are present in between 90 percent and 100 percent of the people who have Graves' disease. Interestingly, other names for this test are the following:

- Anti-thyrotropin
- Anti-TSHR
- Antibodies to TSH receptor
- Thyrotropin-binding inhibitory immunoglobulin) (TBII)
- Thyroid stimulating immunoglobulin

- Thyroid-stimulating hormone receptor (TSH receptor) antibody
- Thyrotropin receptor antibody
- TSH receptor antibody
- TSH receptor-blocking antibody

Thyroid Stimulating Immunoglobulin (TSI)

Thyroid stimulating immunoglobulin (TSI) is a newer test that is used to identify the presence of autoimmune disease in individuals with hyperthyroidism. This test is also called TSH-receptor IgG immunoglobulin test. Abnormally high levels of TSI in your body are predictive of Graves' disease. TSI should be differentiated from other thyroid antibodies such as thyroglobulin antibodies and thyroid-peroxidase antibodies. Studies have revealed that the diagnostic performance of fully automated TSI assay in GD patients is at least comparable to that of current TRAb immunoassays (IMAs), suggesting the possibility of including such assay in rapid and cost-saving diagnostic and monitoring algorithms. Some authors suggest that the TSI assay might be better than the TRAb assay in the initial differential diagnosis of Graves' disease from other thyroid diseases.

Imaging Tests

Thyroid ultrasound supports the diagnosis of Graves' disease as a non-invasive, rapid, and accurate imaging procedure. If a goiter with large nodules is present and/or if radioactive iodine (RAI) therapy is indicated, radionuclide scintigraphy with radioiodine uptake is suggested. In most cases, a positive TSH-R-Ab with a typical ultrasound finding offers a reliable, rapid, and more than sufficient definitive diagnosis of Graves' disease.

Scan of Your Eye Area

In the case of Graves' disease, if an individual is showing either irritation around the eye and socket, or there is a bulging of the eyes, an ultrasound, magnetic resonance imaging (MRI), or computed tomography (CT) scan may be performed to determine the extent of impact the irritation has caused.

Based upon the patient's family history, risk factors, symptoms, and test results, your doctor will determine if the problem is Graves' disease.

Medical Therapies

There are several medical options available to combat Graves' disease. Each option should be considered in light of how far the Graves' disease has progressed.

Beta Blockers (B-Adrenergic Antagonist Drugs)

Beta blockers were originally designed to reduce blood pressure by blocking the effects of the hormone epinephrine, also called adrenaline. It does this by slowing down the number of heartbeats per minute as well opening up blocked vessels. This, in turn, reduces tachycardia, palpitations, tremor, and anxiety. The effects of beta blockers are fast, so it is important for use early in the treatment of Graves' disease. These drugs do not affect thyroid function, release, or synthesis. Beta blockers are not usually used alone for treatment of Graves' disease except for short time frames before and/or after radioactive therapy. Beta blockers should not be used if you have asthma, emphysema, congestive heart failure, bradycardia (slow heartbeat), hypotension (low blood pressure), COPD (chronic obstructive pulmonary disease), or Raynaud's phenomenon.

Anti-thyroid Medication

One of the first options offered is anti-thyroid medications. Anti-thyroid drugs are designed to interfere with the thyroid gland's ability to produce hormones, thereby decreasing hormone production. Unlike other treatments, once they are discontinued, they allow the thyroid to function as usual. Side effects many vary with each drug. These may include nausea, vomiting, heartburn, headache, rash, joint pain, loss of taste, liver failure, or a decrease in disease-fighting white blood cells. Pregnant women should always check with their doctor regarding when they can start on such medications. These drugs can usually be discontinued once a stable normal thyroid balance has been achieved with other therapies.

However, recurrence of hyperthyroidism after a 12 to 18 month course of antithyroid drugs occurs in approximately 50 percent of patients. Being younger than 40 years, having free T4 concentrations that are 40 pmol/L or higher, having TSH-binding inhibitory immunoglobulins that are higher than 6 U/L, and having a goiter size that is equivalent to or larger than WHO grade 2 before the start of treatment with antithyroid drugs increase risk of recurrence. Long-term treatment with antithyroid drugs (for example, 5 to 10 years of treatment) is feasible and associated with fewer recurrences (15 percent) than short-term treatment (for example, 12 to 18 months of treatment). Let's take a closer look at some of these medications.

Glucocorticoids. Glucocorticoids in high doses inhibit the peripheral conversion of T4 to T3. In the treatment of Graves' disease, glucocorticoids decrease T4 secretion by the thyroid gland. How effective this response is or how long it lasts is not known. Use of glucocorticoids is usually not suggested for Graves' disease unless there is major eye or skin involvement or if the patient is in thyroid storm. Short-term use only for these conditions is suggested.

Iodine and iodine-containing compounds. Pharmacologic doses of iodine such as Lugol's solution or saturated solution of potassium iodide (SSKI) work by the following mechanisms:

- Decrease iodine transport into the thyroid

- Inhibit iodine organification and blocks the release of T4 and T3 from the thyroid gland

- Decrease the vascularity of the thyroid in Graves' disease

The effects are only transient, lasting only a few days to weeks. Thyrotoxicosis may return and even worsen. Consequently, iodine therapy is used only short term in preparation for surgery after a normal state has been achieved and maintained with the use of thionamides. Iodine is also used to treat thyroid storm since it can inhibit thyroid hormone immediately.

Oral cholecystographic agents. Oral cholecystographic agents (iodine containing radiocontrast agents), such as iopanoic acid and sodium ipodate, produce a rapid fall in thyroid hormones. They act by inhibition of the peripheral conversion of T4 to T3 and by prevention of thyroid hormone secretion because of the inorganic iodine that is released from the drug. Both iopanoic acid and sodium ipodate because of their rapid onset of action are very effective treatments for Graves' disease. They are not effective for long-term treatment because of the escape of thyroid hormone synthesis from the blocking action of iodine. Furthermore, iopanoic acid and sodium ipodate provide a load of iodine to the thyroid, which makes the using of radioactive iodine not feasible for weeks. Therefore, these drugs are best used for emergency situations for a rapid decrease in thyroid hormone production or prior to surgery.

Perchlorate. Perchlorate works by inhibiting the transport of iodine into the thyroid. Possible side effects include stomach irritation and aplastic anemia. These side effects are somewhat common; therefore, it stops the use of perchlorate as treatment for Graves' disease long-term. Used in conjunction with thionamides, perchlorate has been used successfully for depleting the thyroidal iodine overload in amiodarone-induced hyperthyroidism.

Thionamides. There are three thionamides drugs, methimazole (MMI), carbimazole, and propylthiouracil (PTU), which are effective in their treatment of Graves'. Thionamides do not block the release of preformed thyroid hormone. They inhibit thyroid peroxidase, blocking the making of T3 and T4. Consequently, it takes 1 to 6 weeks for the thyroid hormones that are already stored and the iodine that is stored to be depleted and the patient to have total relief of symptoms and normalization of thyroid studies. Large goiters with large deposits of thyroid hormone may show a delayed response to thionamides. Thionamides represent the treatment of choice in pregnant women, during lactation, in children and adolescents, and in preparation for radioiodine therapy or thyroidectomy (removal of the thyroid gland).

The main problem with the use of thionamides is that there is a high relapse rate when the medications are stopped. The recurrence rate is 50 to 80 percent depending on the length of follow-up. Most relapses occur within 3 to 6 months but can occur much later. Remission rates have decreased over the last decade, perhaps due to an increased iodine supply in the diet of the average American. Relapse after treatment suggests that another form of treatment may be necessary. Some patients become hypothyroid after therapy.

Mild side effects have been reported in 1 to 15 percent of patients that take thionamides, such as:

- Hives (urticaria)
- Itching (pruritus)
- Joint pain (arthralgias)
- Slightly elevated liver enzymes
- Skin rash

Severe side effects of thionamides are rare and require prompt discontinuation of the medication. These side effects include:

- Cholestatic necrotic hepatitis

- Decrease of white blood cells (agranulocytosis)
- Inflammation of blood vessels (vasculitis)

- Lupus-like syndrome
- Toxic hepatitis

Thionamides can serve as a long-term therapy or as a bridge to I-131 ablation or thyroidectomy (thyroid surgery), with the goal of normalizing thyroid function and preventing exacerbation of hyperthyroidism after I-131 ablation or avoiding surgical risks associated with uncontrolled hyperthyroidism. Because Graves' disease remits in up to 30 percent of patients treated with thionamides, these medications can be used as the initial treatment, with ablation or thyroidectomy performed if remission does not occur. Once medical therapy is discontinued, relapse occurs in 30 percent to 70 percent of people, mostly within the first year. After discontinuation, thyroid function should be monitored by your healthcare provider on a regular basis. Contact your physician if symptoms recur.

Radioactive Iodine Therapy

Radioactive iodine ablation of the thyroid gland is the most common treatment of Graves' disease in the United States. It is contraindicated in pregnancy or nursing. Moderate to severe Graves' eye disease is a relative contraindication, especially in patients who smoke, because radioactive iodine may exacerbate the eye disease. In mild cases of Graves' ophthalmopathy, radioactive iodine ablation can be performed together with steroid therapy. Nonradioactive iodine impedes radioactive iodine uptake by iodide transporter; therefore, exposure to large amounts of nonradioactive iodine (such as iodinated contrast and amiodarone) should be avoided within three months before radioactive iodine ablation. Pregnancy should be ruled out within 48 hours before radioactive iodine ablation and avoided for six months thereafter. A thionamide should be discontinued at least five days before the treatment but can be restarted three to five days after to maintain control of thyroid function, because it may take up to twelve weeks to achieve the full effect of radioactive iodine.

With this therapy, a radioactive form of iodine is orally taken. As the reactive iodine is absorbed, the low-level radiation is enough to destroy the overactive thyroid cells causing the thyroid to shrink and produce less hormones. The treatment is taken over several weeks. With the decrease in thyroid hormones, the symptoms of disease are lessened.

Because this treatment involves destroying thyroid cells, it will likely have an effect on the amount of thyroid hormones produced in the future. Most people develop permanent hypothyroidism between two and six months after radioactive iodine ablation and require thyroid hormone replacement. Free T4 and free T3 should be measured four to eight weeks after ablation; if hyperthyroidism persists, these indices should be monitored every four to six weeks and thyroid hormone replacement started in the early stages of hypothyroidism.

Surgery

In serious cases, surgically removing part or the whole thyroid gland may be considered. With the partial or whole removal, a patient's levels of thyroid hormones must be carefully monitored. If the entire or partial gland is removed, individuals will normally be required to take thyroid medication for the remainder of their lives. This treatment option is preferred in patients with goiter-induced compressive symptoms and in patients with contraindications to radioactive iodine ablation or thionamides. Besides general anesthesia risk, thyroidectomy carries a risk of inadvertently injuring the parathyroid glands and recurrent laryngeal nerves.

Thyroid Eye Disease (TED) Treatments

All patients with TED must be assessed for disease activity and severity to determine the best course of action. Risk factor modification begins with smoking cessation and attaining euthyroid—a normally functioning thyroid gland—status.

- For mild symptoms of TED, patients can use over-the-counter artificial tears during the day and lubricating gels at night to avoid corneal damage caused by exposure and for relief.

- For moderate to severe symptoms, your doctor may recommend the following treatments:

Corrective lens. In cases of double vision because of Graves' disease, or as a side effect of surgery for Graves', glasses containing prism lenses may be prescribed to normalize vision. The outcome of vision improvement may vary from patient to patient.

Corticosteroids. Treatment with corticosteroids, such as prednisone, will help reduce swelling behind your eyeballs. Side effects may include fluid retention, weight gain, elevated blood sugar levels, increased blood pressure, and mood swings. Corticosteroids are the first-line treatment for moderate to severe symptoms. But often a multifaceted approach with the addition of orbital decompression may be needed.

Dry eyes. As soon as you begin to experience dry eyes or a sensation of grit or irritation in the eye, start to use artificial tears or eye drops to prevent any scratching of the cornea. Check with your doctor for a brand recommendation. You may also use eye covers at night to keep the eyes shut and prevent them from becoming dry.

Eyelid surgery. This procedure may be performed to restore the eyelid to an appropriate position, allowing a patient to either close their eyes or to reduce sagging eyelid tissue to improve appearance.

Orbital decompression surgery. In this operation, the surgeon removes the bone between the eye socket and your sinuses, providing more room for the eyes to move back to their original position. This treatment should be considered when the pressure on the optic nerve may lead to blindness. Possible complications include double vision.

OTHER MEDICAL TREATMENTS

Once a diagnosis of Graves' disease has been confirmed, there are a number of therapies available to treat the condition. With this disease, patients should seek to reduce the level of their body's autoimmune response.

- Begin by avoiding all gluten as a lifetime change in your diet. Also avoid all foods you are allergic to.

- In addition, consider going on a detox diet that pulls out inflammatory foods, which may alleviate thyroid symptoms. (See "Detoxification" on page 63).

- Next achieving optimal gastrointestinal function may decrease or resolve your symptoms. (See Chapter 11 on page 235) Have your healthcare provider order a gut health test and then follow all of the directions that they suggest in order to improve the health of your GI tract.

- Furthermore, and very importantly, discuss with your healthcare provider starting low-dose naltrexone (LDN) as a lifetime therapy. (See page 70.)

PERSONALIZED MEDICINE TREATMENTS

While there are no natural short-cuts for treating Graves' disease, there are a number of natural treatment options to consider. These must be used in conjunction with standard medical treatment along with avoiding gluten, fixing the gut, and LDN. Before starting any, each natural option should be discussed with your healthcare provider.

Acupuncture

Acupuncture, the use of small needles strategically placed in the skin, has been used as a treatment in China for thousands of years. Studies in China have shown it effective in treating Graves' disease.

Cold Packs

By placing ice packs over the thyroid gland, found at the base of your neck, three times a day, you can reduce swelling. The cold will also help slow down the function of the thyroid gland.

Diet

Eat foods that are good for you. Whole fruits, vegetables, and nuts top the list. In addition, a high protein diet has been shown to be mildly effective against mild Graves' disease. These foods contain goitrogens, a naturally occurring chemical, which has been shown to prevent or make it more difficult for utilization of iodine. In so doing, they block thyroid synthesis. These goitrogenic foods include:

- Almonds
- Broccoli
- Brussels sprouts
- Cabbage
- Cassava root
- Cauliflower
- Kohlrabi
- Millet
- Mustard
- Peaches
- Peanuts
- Pine nuts
- Rapeseeds
- Rutabagas
- Soybeans
- Sweet potatoes
- Turnip

However, it is important to understand these foods cannot be reliably used in place of medications in the treatment of Graves' disease, since their goitrogen content is low. Furthermore, cooking inactivates the goitrogens. Likewise, no substantial documentation is available to show that dietary goitrogens interfere with thyroid function if the patient has adequate levels of iodine. Also, foods that are high in iodine content, such as seaweeds, should be avoided.

Studies have shown that people should eat foods that contain flavonoids since they decrease serum T4 and inhibit both the conversion of T4 to T3 and 5′deiodinase activity. Food such as fruits and vegetables of yellow, orange, red, and purple color, such as blueberries, purple grapes, and cherries, contain flavonoids.

Limiting Your Food Choices

When treating Graves' disease, you should avoid consuming any food or drinks that will interfere with normal thyroid function.

Avoid caffeine. Caffeine can increase the severity of many Graves' disease symptoms, such as rapid heart rate, anxiety, and tremors. By eliminating products such as soda, coffee, tea, and chocolate from your diet, you can control some of these persistent issues.

Avoid foods that you are allergic to. While it may be easy to identify foods and avoid the foods you are allergic to, there are people who have hidden food allergies that they may not be aware of—from dairy (containing lactose) to soy to wheat (containing gluten) products. Many of these food allergies can aggravate Graves' symptoms. Make sure you are aware of all the foods you may be allergic to.

Avoid foods with high iodine content. It is wise to avoid foods containing a high level of iodine, such as sea vegetables, iodized salt, and some fish and seafood, since iodine can affect the overproduction of the thyroid hormones. In addition, betadine washes, and iodine-containing medications, such as amiodarone and radiographic dyes, should be avoided if possible. Do not discontinue any medication without working with your physician. Iodine excess may be a problem particularly in people that take iodine without having their levels measured. The use of iodine in patients that have Graves' disease is unpredictable and it is not suggested for usage.

Avoid heavily processed foods. Cut down or stop consuming foods that are heavily processed, salted, and/or sugared. Also, make sure to consume foods low in iodine. Find a healthful diet that you can stick to.

Exercise and Light-weight Training

While exercise is good for so many healthful reasons, when it comes to Graves' disease it can help in two ways. When the issue is weight gain, burning carbs through exercise can help keep pounds off. Secondly, with Graves' there is a tendency to have brittle bones. Light-weight training can strengthen bones as well as strengthen leg muscles for better balance and to prevent falls from occurring.

Reducing Stress

Studies have shown that stress may trigger or worsen Graves' disease symptoms. By learning how to control stress in your life, you can avoid those stress-related hormones that may interfere in your healing process. Find the activity you enjoy most that you can relax doing—from taking long walks and hot baths to learning yoga exercises. This simple change in your life can make a difference. Have your healthcare provider measure your stress hormone, cortisol, by salivary testing to determine if stress is playing a major role in this disease process.

Stop Smoking

Research has shown that smoking can increase the symptoms associated with Graves' disease—especially those who suffer from Graves' thyroid eye disease. In addition, it can affect the outcome of various thyroid treatments. Giving up smoking may not be easy, but it may be a lot easier to do knowing it's something that can help you beat the disease.

Nutritional Supplements

Another option for people with Graves' is taking nutritional supplements. However, taking nutritional supplements alone may not be enough to overcome this thyroid disease. There are a number of factors that should be considered when trying to improve your thyroid health, and taking certain nutritional supplements can be beneficial.

Calcium citrate. Calcium metabolism may be changed in hyperthyroidism where patients with Graves' disease have an increased risk of developing osteoporosis. Supplementing with calcium may be beneficial.

Coenzyme Q-10. Like a vitamin, this substance is a cofactor in the electron-transport chain, which is the energy producing cycle in the body. Q-10 levels have been shown to be low in adults and children with hyperthyroidism. Studies have also shown that coenzyme Q-10 levels may return to normal after treatment of hyperthyroidism with conventional therapies. It may be helpful to supplement with Q-10 in people with Graves' disease that have cardiac disease and also in individuals with long-standing uncorrected hyperthyroidism.

L-carnitine. This amino acid is used for the transport of long-chain fatty acids into the mitochondria. L-carnitine is an antagonist of thyroid hormone in peripheral tissues by inhibiting thyroid hormone entry into the nucleus of the cells. One study conducted over 6 months used carnitine in patients with hyperthyroidism. Patients taking L-carnitine improved their symptoms and liver profiles, but the patients that did not take L-carnitine were worse. The form of L-carnitine used should be L-carnitine alone or the acetic or propionic acid form and not the D-form. Also, L-carnitine is cleared through the kidneys so it should only be considered in individuals with normal kidney function. You cannot take L-carnitine if you have an elevated TMAO level. Have your doctor measure your TMAO level, which is a fasting blood study, before starting this nutrient.

Selenium. People with Graves' commonly have low selenium (a trace mineral) levels. In fact, selenium deficiency alters the conversion of T4 to T3 in peripheral tissues such as the kidney and the liver. One study found men fed low selenium diets had their serum T3 levels increase. Selenium is one of the supplements that should be considered as a therapy for mild hyperthyroidism in people that are not high in selenium or selenium toxic. Eating Brazil nuts and other foods that are high in selenium is also helpful.

In a number of studies, it was found that a deficiency of selenium was found in a number of patients suffering from Graves' thyroid eye disease. When put on a daily dosage of 100 micrograms of selenium selenite twice daily for 6 months, there was an observable improvement of symptoms associated with mild TED. Additionally, the same amount of selenium taken by Graves' patients showed a significant decrease in their thyroid peroxidase antibody levels—one of the culprits that trigger the thyroid's overproduction of hormones. Moreover, selenium supplementation in Graves' orbitopathy is associated with an improvement of quality of life and eye involvement, as well as delayed progression of ocular disorders.

Vitamin A. Given in large doses, this antioxidant has an inhibitory effect on the thyroid gland. Vitamin A supplementation has been shown to decrease the symptoms of Graves' disease. The exact mechanism by, which vitamin A works is unknown. If you smoke, then do not consider this therapy, since large doses of vitamin A in smokers may be linked to an increased risk of developing lung cancer.

Vitamin C (Ascorbic acid). Animal studies have shown that thyroid hormone in excess can reduce ascorbic acid levels in the serum, blood, liver, adrenal glands, thymus, and kidney. Studies in human trials in patients with hyperthyroidism have also shown an increase in excretion of ascorbic acid. Furthermore, trials have shown that the medications thiourea and thiouracil also lower ascorbic acid levels. Consequently, supplementation with vitamin C is suggested in patients with hyperthyroidism. Supplementation does not affect the course of the disease, but it may decrease the symptoms and metabolic effects.

Vitamin E. This vitamin may be protective against oxidative damage caused by Graves' disease. In an animal study, animals with hyperthyroidism were given vitamin E, which helped to prevent the lipid peroxidation that is associated with hyperthyroidism. Human studies have shown that individuals with hyperthyroidism have low vitamin E levels. Consequently, supplementation with vitamin E is suggested.

Zinc. Red blood cell (RBC) zinc levels are lower in patients with Graves' disease since zinc needs are increased because of greater urinary zinc excretion in this disease process. Therapy with anti-thyroid medications has been shown to normalize RBC zinc levels 2 months after free T3 and free T4 have been normalized.

Herbs

There are a number of botanical supplements that may be helpful in some patients with Graves' disease. It is always advisable to work with a trained professional when using such herbal supplementation.

Bugleweed. The German Commission E, Germany's equivalent to the FDA, recognizes the use of bugleweed for mild hyperthyroid conditions associated with the dysfunction of the nervous system based on pharmacologic studies. Activity is mediated by a reduction in TSH, T4, and inhibition of the conversion of T4 tp T3. Bugleweed also inhibits the receptor-binding and biological activity of Graves' immunoglobulins. However, be aware that in rare situations high dosages have resulted in thyroid enlargement and sudden discontinuation has increased disease symptoms.

Club moss. This herb has a long history of use for hyperthyroidism, like bugleweed. Animal studies using club moss have shown its ability to block TSH activity at the receptor level, block the release of TSH from the thyroid, and suppress the iodine pump. It can also inhibit the peripheral T4-deiodination and conversion to T3.

Emblica officinalis. Animal studies using Emblica officinalis are promising. It was shown to reduce T3 and T4 concentrations by a significant amount. Human trials need to be done.

Ginger. It has been found that ginger has a positive effect on thyroid function. Ginger contains magnesium, which has been proven to be a key factor in controlling thyroid disease. Since it aids in regulating inflammation, it is also considered to protect against thyroid conditions that are caused by inflammation. Ginger can be used in various ways. Fresh ginger root can be added when cooking or baking in the diced or powder form. In pill form, start with one capsule, twice a day.

Lemon balm. Lemon balm has calming effects on the nervous system and has been used since ancient times for this issue. Lab studies have confirmed lemon balm's ability to block TSH receptors and inhibit both binding of bovine TSH to human thyroid tissue and binding of auto-antibodies in Graves' disease. It is usually combined with bugleweed to treat Graves' disease. Studies show that this herb is helpful in lowering the production of thyroid hormones when given in injection form. More studies need to be done on the oral form.

Milk Thistle. Milk thistle is another natural therapy for the treatment of Graves' disease and is usually taken in supplement form for this purpose. It contains a flavonoid called silymarin, which contains powerful antioxidant properties that are beneficial in the treatment of this disorder. It also may be helpful for treating eye problems caused by Graves' disease.

Motherwort. This is used traditionally to treat anxiety, depression, heart palpitations, and tachycardia (heart racing). Therefore, it may be good for the relief of symptoms of Graves' disease. It can be used with bugleweed. The German Commission E supports the use of motherwort for the treatment of cardiac disorders associated with anxiety and for the symptomatic relief of mild hyperthyroidism.

Turmeric. Turmeric is an herb that has been used for thousands of years. Like ginger, it can be beneficial in treating inflammation. It has anti-inflammatory properties, which help to treat thyroid dysfunctions such as Graves' disease. You can add turmeric when cooking or it can be taken in capsule form. Follow dosage directions on the package.

There are also botanical medicines that contain flavonoids, such as hawthorne berry, astragalus, ginkgo biloba, licorice, and chamomile that may be helpful therapies in Graves' disease.

OUTCOME (PROGNOSIS)

There are various factors that must be considered when treating Graves' disease: a patient's age, history of hyperthyroidism or Graves' disorder in their family, past and present health status, how serious their Graves' disease is, and their willingness to get better. For many patients with mild to moderate Graves' disease, their condition responds well to treatment. When they also have thyroid eye disease, both conditions must be treated simultaneously. Mild to moderate TED also responds well to treatments. Serious cases of TED may require additional eye surgery. Reversing the condition may take time, however the emphasis should be on maintaining a decent quality of life until it happens.

Thyroid surgery, radioactive iodine, or other medical treatments will commonly cause an underactive thyroid (hypothyroidism). Therefore, it is important to monitor your thyroid hormone levels to avoid the many effects of hypothyroidism. When this happens, to keep your thyroid hormone level in balance, you will normally be required to take thyroid replacement. This may only be necessary until your thyroid is fully functioning or it may be needed for the rest of your life. As long as you are getting the correct dosage of thyroid hormone replacement, you should be able to avoid the symptoms.

CONCLUSION

As you have read, Graves' disease is the most common form of hyperthyroidism. Unfortunately, it can go undetected for years, masquerading as a host of other disorders. Once you have identified the problem as Graves', there is a great deal that can be done to reverse the condition. Of course, the earlier it is caught, the better the outcome. Still, knowing what your best options are and being able to participate in your return to health are important aspects of the healing process.

6

Thyroid Disorders Associated with Hyperthyroidism and Thyrotoxicosis

As we have seen in previous chapters, there are several causes and treatments related to hyperthyroidism and thyrotoxicosis. In the same way, there are various medical conditions that are created by, or associated with, hyperthyroidism and thyrotoxicosis. Many of these disorders come with their own set of symptoms, health issues, and treatments. If you believe that you may be suffering from an overproduction of thyroid hormones, this chapter should provide you with a basic understanding of the remainder of the most common disorders related to this condition. Any form of thyroiditis can be associated with a thyrotoxic phase (hyperthyroidism) because the disruption of thyroid follicles can result in an increased release of stored iodothyronines. The thyrotoxic phase may be followed by transient or permanent hypothyroidism. The uptake of radioiodine is very low or absent in the thyrotoxic phase and serum thyroglobulin levels are high.

AUTONOMOUSLY FUNCTIONING THYROID NODULES (AFTN)/TOXIC ADENOMA

An autonomously functioning thyroid nodule (AFTN) is a well-defined mass of thyroid cells that grow either on the surface or within the thyroid gland. They may appear as patchy areas, a single nodule, or multiple nodules. When they appear as multiple nodules, this condition is referred to as Plummer's disease or toxic adenoma. These nodules are capable of producing and secreting thyroid hormone independent of stimulation by TSH. Because these nodules can produce more thyroid hormones than the body requires, this condition can lead to hyperthyroidism.

About 7 percent of people have some sort of abnormal growth on their thyroid. A thyroid adenoma is one type of growth and is estimated to occur in 3 percent to 4 percent of people. Thyroid adenomas are more common in women than men.

There are two types of autonomously functioning thyroid nodules: warm and hot. The term *warm* is given to nodules that do not produce sufficient amounts of hormones to disrupt the production of TSH. As a warm nodule enlarges in size, it may begin to produce more thyroid hormones. In addition, it may slow down the uptake activity of the surrounding thyroid tissue. When it produces an excess amount of thyroid hormone and begins to affect the surrounding tissue, it is referred to as a *hot* nodule. This condition can bring on hyperthyroidism. As it becomes bigger in size, it can also be referred to as toxic.

Only a small number—5 to 10 percent—of solitary thyroid nodules are toxic. A toxic adenoma is a monoclonal, autonomously functioning thyroid nodule (AFTN) that produces supraphysiological (greater than normally present in the body) amounts of T4 and/or T3 resulting in suppression (lower than normal levels) of serum TSH. The function of the surrounding normal thyroid tissue is often, but not always, suppressed. This varies depending on the country the individual is from. For example, the numbers are higher in Europe. The development of hyperthyroidism occurs mainly in nodules that are greater than 3 centimeters with a minimal volume of 16 milliliters on an ultrasound of the thyroid.

It is important to also point out that just finding a nodule on the thyroid gland does not mean the growth is malignant. In fact, these nodules are commonly benign. Each year there are over 1.2 million patients who are diagnosed with thyroid nodules. Many of these nodules are ruled out as benign using an ultrasound scan. Furthermore, of the 525,000 to 600,000 nodules that are biopsied every year, only 10 percent are found to be malignant. (See Chapter 18 on page 297 for more information on malignant nodules.)

RISK FACTORS

Risk factors include iodine deficiency, head and neck irradiation, and family history of thyroid nodules.

SIGNS AND SYMPTOMS

The signs and symptoms of patients with toxic adenoma or AFTN are the same as they are for hyperthyroidism. (See Chapter 4 on page 75.) Hyperphagia (excessive eating), weight loss, sweating, heat intolerance, and nervousness are the most common.

TESTS

There are tests available to determine whether you have an autonomously functioning thyroid nodule.

Physical Examination

Normally, a physician can see some of the more pronounced signs, such a lump in the neck, thyroid enlargement, or signs of tremors, which can indicate hyperthyroidism. Your healthcare provider will also palpate your thyroid gland to see if it is enlarged.

Blood Tests

Unfortunately, measuring the level of the thyroid-stimulating hormone (TSH) in your blood may not indicate whether you have AFTN. Because AFTN may not affect the TSH level, you will need an ultrasound scan to detect this condition.

Thyroid Ultrasound Scan

Sound waves are used to create a visual image of the thyroid. This is done when a small wand-like instrument is moved along the skin in front of the thyroid gland. The black and white image seen on a computer screen will show whether the node is composed of a solid mass of cells or a cyst containing blood or pus. If it is a solid node, further testing needs to be done to determine if the mass is benign or malignant.

Fine Needle Aspiration (FNA)

If a node is found, a fine needle aspiration is taken. The skin above the node is numbed, and a thin needle is inserted into the node to remove cells and fluid for review. These samples are then sent to a laboratory, where a pathologist examines them under a microscope to determine the exact nature of the cells. The pathologist writes up a report on his findings and sends back the report to the ordering physician.

TREATMENT

No treatment of a *hot* nodule is needed as long as you have normal thyroid function. Thyroid labs are usually repeated every 6 months since there is a concern for potential progression to hyperthyroidism. The possibility of a warm nodule being cancerous is there, so it is evaluated the same way a *cold* nodule is. (A cold nodule is a thyroid nodule with a much lower uptake of radioactive iodine than the surrounding nodules during a radioactive iodine uptake scan, while a hot nodule shows an increase in radioactive uptake.) There are a number of effective treatments for AFTN. Your options may be based on the nature of your AFTN and the state of your health. Treatment with antithyroid drugs is used infrequently as it requires long-term therapy, and a relapse will almost invariably occur after discontinuation of the medication. However, usually the individual is treated preoperatively with antithyroid drugs and beta-blockers to minimize symptoms before surgery.

Surgery

If necessary, removing the node surgically may be a strong consideration. Surgical excision permits the achievement of rapid and permanent control of hyperthyroidism with a very low operative complication rate. The disadvantage of a surgical approach includes the risks of general anesthesia and the potential complications of thyroid surgery. This therapy is very successful, and a small number of people become hypothyroid afterwards. However, in a recent study by Bolusani, evaluating 105 patients with solitary autonomous nodules, the cumulative incidence of hypothyroidism was 11 percent at 1 year, 33 percent at 5 years, and 49 percent at 10 years. Therefore, your doctor will follow you long-term to determine your thyroid function.

Radioactive Iodine Therapy (RAI)

With this therapy, a radioactive form of iodine (131 iodine) is orally taken by the patient. As the reactive iodine is absorbed, the low-level radiation is enough to destroy the overactive thyroid cells causing the thyroid to shrink and produce less hormones. The treatment is taken over several weeks. This is a widely used therapeutic modality for individuals with toxic adenomas. Patients may become hypothyroid more commonly if they have positive thyroid antibodies. A small number of people may develop Graves' disease from radioactive iodine.

Percutaneous Ethanol Injections (PEI)

This treatment or radiofrequency ablation may be used when surgery and radioactive iodine cannot be done. It involves injecting ethanol, an alcohol solution, into the nodule. The injection results in necrosis and thrombosis of small vessels. This therapy requires a series of injections. This treatment has been shown to be safe and effective, especially with nodules that contain fluid. Side effects include local pain and, in rare cases, recurrent nerve damage. In studies evaluating the outcomes at 12 or 30 months, about 85 percent of patients were euthyroid. Results of ethanol injection in relatively large AFTNs (diameter 3 to 4 cm) are also favorable, particularly in patients with subclinical hyperthyroidism.

Radiofrequency Ablation (RFA)

In this procedure, a needle electrode is inserted into the nodule through the skin. An electrical current produced by radio waves is used to heat up a small area contained within the nodule. This results in the destruction (ablation) of the nodule.

OUTCOME (PROGNOSIS)

The vast majority of AFTN treatments are highly effective. Side effects may range from hypothyroidism to Graves' disease. Where no serious symptoms are observed, your physician may ask that you come in for frequent check-ups to observe the AFTN.

MULTINODULAR GOITER (MNG): NONTOXIC AND TOXIC

Multinodular goiter occurs when several nodules are present on a partially or entirely enlarged thyroid gland. Most goiters are small and produce no or few symptoms. If the goiter consists of more than one autonomous thyroid nodule, or one or more autonomous nodules together with one or more nonautonomous solid, cystic, or mixed (solid and cystic) nodules, or numerous small autonomous areas, it may be associated with a spectrum of hyperthyroidism ranging from subclinical hyperthyroidism to severe thyrotoxicosis. Autonomous nodules appear as hyperactive (hot or warm) and nonautonomous nodules as hypoactive (cold), or normoactive, on nuclear medicine thyroid scintigraphy. When symptoms are present, they are usually related to the growth and function of the thyroid.

There are two forms of this type of goiter, nontoxic and toxic multinodular goiter. Toxic multinodular goiter (MNG) is a hormonally active multinodular goiter where a person exhibits symptoms of hyperthyroidism. People that have a *nontoxic multinodular goiter* usually do not have any signs or symptoms and may have normal thyroid function. A nontoxic multinodular goiter is usually slow to evolve and most often occurs in the elderly. They are prevalent particularly in areas of the world that are iodine deficient. Therefore, studies have shown that populations that regularly consume iodized salt, or eat foods that are rich in iodine, have much fewer causes of MNG than those communities that do not. Individuals with nontoxic multinodular goiter may become hyperthyroid. Less commonly they become hypothyroid. The hyperthyroidism may develop insidiously. Commonly there is a long time of subclinical (undetected) hyperthyroidism where the person will have low TSH and normal free T4 and T3. The hyperthyroidism is due to the growth of the goiter and an associated increase in the mass of autonomously hormone-producing cells. The hyperthyroidism may also be due to use of iodine supplements or iodine containing drugs, such as amiodarone or dye. Transition from nontoxic goiter to toxic goiter may be part of the development of the disease. The timeframe between when the goiter is nontoxic and becomes toxic is unknown.

In contrast, the most common cause of *diffuse toxic goiter*, is Graves' disease, which is the most common cause of hyperthyroidism in the United States and affects 1 in 200 people. It usually affects people between 30 and 50 years of age but can occur in any age group. Graves' is 7 to 10 times more common in females than in males. For more information on Graves' disease see Chapter 5 on page 97.

RISK FACTORS

The risk factors for multinodular goiter are not clearly understood, however there are a number of circumstances that researchers believe can lead to this condition.

Genetics

Genetics seem to play a role in some patients. However, it may require one or more triggers to initiate the condition, which are listed below.

Age

Statistics indicate that MNG occurs most often in people over the age of 60 if it is nontoxic. In individuals with diffuse toxic goiter, the most common age group is between 30 and 50 years.

Gender

Females are at higher risk to develop MNG than males.

Environmental Conditions

Potentially any number of heavy metals and pollutants may build up and trigger this disease process.

SIGNS AND SYMPTOMS

The majority of multinodular goiters are nontoxic, show no symptoms, and are only discovered during a physical exam. However, toxic multinodular goiters may show any of the following signs and symptoms:

- Enlargement of the thyroid gland during pregnancy
- Gradual development of hyperthyroidism
- Hoarseness
- Difficulty swallowing

Horner's syndrome

Signs and symptoms of Horner's syndrome include decreased pupil size, a drooping eyelid, and decreased sweating on the affected side of the face. This condition is rare.

- Iodine-induced thyrotoxicosis
- Obstruction of the superior vena cava (superior vena cava obstruction syndrome)
- Obstruction of the thoracic inlet by extending the arms over the head (Pemberton's sign)
- Occasional cough and difficulty swallowing
- Phrenic nerve palsy (rare)
- Recurrent nerve palsy (rare)
- Slowly growing nodular anterior neck mass
- Sudden pain or enlargement secondary to bleeding (hemorrhage)
- Upper airway obstruction, shortness of breath, and tracheal compression

CAUSES

Goiters can materialize when the thyroid gland produces either too much or too little thyroid hormone. In the case of a nontoxic multinodular goiter, the enlargement can come about with a normal production of thyroid hormone.

Iodine Deficiency

Studies have shown that populations that regularly consume iodized salt have much fewer cases of MNG than those communities that do not since iodine deficiency or impairment of iodine metabolism by the thyroid gland, perhaps due to congenital biochemical defects, may be an important mechanism leading to increases in TSH secretion.

Cigarette Smoking

The organic chemical thiocyanate is generated when you smoke, which may cause a goiter.

Medications

Medications such as lithium, iodides, interferon-alpha, amiodarone may increase your risk. Do not discontinue taking any medication without consulting your physician.

Diet

A diet high in natural goitrogens—substances that suppress the function of the thyroid gland by interfering with iodine intake may result in a goiter such as:

- Broccoli
- Cauliflower
- Kale
- Brussels sprouts
- Mustard greens
- Radishes
- Peaches
- Soy-based foods
- Peanuts
- Spinach
- Strawberries

While many of these foods are healthy for you, like anything else, it is important not to eat too much of one single food. Moderation is the key to health!

Selenium Deficiency

Studies have shown that low selenium levels are a cause of MNG. Have your healthcare provider order your selenium level to determine if you need to take a selenium supplement. This is one mineral that you can become toxic in, therefore it is important to have measured.

Autoimmune Disorders

A history of an autoimmune disorder such as Hashimoto's or Graves' disease increases the risk of the development of this disorder.

Iron Deficiency

Low levels of iron or suboptimal levels of iron have been shown to be associated with multinodular goiter. Have your healthcare provider measure your iron levels and supplement if needed. You should have a repeat iron level done in 90 days. Iron is a substance that if levels are elevated in your body, it increases your risk of other diseases, including heart disease.

DIAGNOSIS

There are quite a few tests available to determine whether you have a multinodular goiter (MNG).

Physical Examination

Normally, a physician can see some of the more pronounced signs, such a lump in the neck, thyroid enlargement, or signs of respiratory distress, which can indicate MNG.

Blood Tests

The blood test is the most common test and plays an important role in diagnosing thyroid disease and treating thyroid conditions. Several blood tests will be done to determine if you are suffering from MNG. The primary evaluation consists of a complete thyroid profile, including TSH, free T3, free T4, reverse T3, and thyroid antibodies.

Imaging Tests

Laboratory tests are not always accurate in diagnosing a dysfunction in the thyroid. Sometimes more tests are ordered. Imaging tests are administered for a diagnosis of various thyroid disorders. These can include an ultrasound, CT scan, MRI, scintigraphy (used for diagnosis test in nuclear medicine), or a PET scan. Radioactive iodine uptake or a combination of thyroid ultrasound with TSH-receptor antibodies is the most common testing performed.

Fine Needle Aspiration (FNA)

If MNG is found, a fine needle aspiration is taken. The skin above the node is numbed and a thin needle is inserted into the area to remove cells for review. These samples are then sent to a laboratory, where a pathologist examines them under a microscope to determine the exact nature of the cells. The pathologist writes up a report on his findings and sends back the report to the ordering physician.

TREATMENT

Treatment of a nontoxic multinodular goiter depends on the symptoms. Nontoxic nodular thyroid disease is common. Many of these goiters do not cause major symptoms and may not need to be treated after proven non-cancerous. Treatment should be considered in the following cases:

- Cosmetic complaints

- Large goiter or progressive growth of entire gland or individual nodules

- Marked neck disfigurement

- Overt or subclinical hyperthyroidism
- Signs of cervical compression

There is no perfect treatment protocol for multinodular goiter. Treatments that are used include thionamides, which are antithyroid medications, levothyroxine, surgery, and radioactive iodine. In today's world, surgery and radioactive therapy are the most commonly used therapeutic modalities.

Antithyroid Medication

Antithyroid medications, also called thionamides, are used if a nodular goiter is complicated by hyperthyroidism. These drugs stop the production of TSH. Remission is rare, and usually treatment is indicated for life. Further growth may occur. Thionamides are also indicated before surgery to lower operative risk. To decrease the risk of making the hyperthyroidism worse, thionamides are also suggested before radioactive iodine treatment.

Thyroid hormone therapy with levothyroxine for suppression of the pituitary TSH secretion has been used in the past, but since the natural progression of the goiter is to progress into hyperthyroidism, levothyroxine therapy is no longer suggested. Antithyroid medications can control hyperthyroidism, but do not induce remission of hyperthyroidism associated with toxic adenoma or toxic multinodular goiter. Therefore, radioactive iodine ablation and thyroidectomy are the main treatment options for these conditions. Thyroidectomy is favored if a nodule or goiter causes compressive symptoms. Antithyroid medications may be used for long-term treatment in select patients who refuse ablation or who have a contraindication to thyroidectomy.

Surgery

The goal of surgery is to remove all thyroid tissue with a nodular appearance. Some surgeons remove part of the thyroid and other surgeons suggest the entire thyroid be taken out to prevent a recurrence. In the case of toxic nodular goiter, thyroid function is usually normalized more commonly with surgery than with radioactive iodine. Thionamides are not needed after surgery. Complications occasionally occur with surgery to the thyroid gland, which may include infection, bleeding, vocal cord paralysis, or hypoparathyroidism. Rarely other complications may occur.

It is the preferred treatment in people who are unable to tolerate antithyroid medications or radioactive iodine, or in patients with compressive symptoms.

Radioactive Iodine (RAI)

Radioactive iodine is considered by many physicians as a safe treatment in many cases of hyperthyroidism, particularly in older people. It has a lower cost and less complication rate. Radioactive iodine is administered in liquid or capsule forms. You must discontinue all iodine-containing medication and be on an iodine restricted diet to ensure effective uptake of RAI. Anti-thyroid medication must be discontinued before the use of RAI and can be resumed after a week of administering radioactive iodine if needed. Twenty to 40 percent of people will need a second dose of radioactive iodine. It causes the thyroid gland to shrink. It usually shrinks the same amount in toxic or nontoxic goiters. One possible complication of radioactive iodine treatment is radiation thyroiditis (inflammation of the thyroid gland), which is treated with steroids or salicylates. Another possible complication with radioactive iodine treatment is Graves' disease, an autoimmune type of hyperthyroidism, which is seen in about 5 percent of people. Worsening of thyroid-associated ophthalmopathy (eye disease) may also occur.

If you have positive thyroid antibodies before treatment, the risk of Graves' disease is more common. This can also be seen after surgery and in subacute thyroiditis. Enlargement of the thyroid gland has not been seen after therapy. The risk of developing permanent hypothyroidism after radioactive iodine in multinodular goiters is from 14 percent to 58 percent within 5 to 8 years. This occurs more commonly in patients that have smaller goiter size to begin with and patients that have positive thyroid antibodies. The ability for radioactive iodine to work in multinodular goiter is decreased if there are a lot of nodules. Possible side effects of the treatment are hyperthyroidism and toxicity if larger doses are used. The absolute contraindications of this therapy are pregnancy, breastfeeding, and severe uncontrolled thyrotoxicosis. Follow-up is lifelong since you can develop a recurrence or hypothyroidism and need prompt treatment.

OUTCOMES (PROGNOSIS)

A multinodular goiter that causes no apparent symptoms is unlikely to cause problems over time, however, as mentioned above, it should be checked regularly by a physician. In the case of toxic multinodular goiters, immediate treatment should be undertaken. Individuals with diffuse toxic goiter, especially due to Graves' disease, are expected to become hypothyroid during the natural course of their disease regardless of treatment. Prolonged thyrotoxicosis may cause ventricular thickening and, therefore, an increased risk of cardiac mortality (death due to heart disease). Treatment with RAI is done with the aim of permanent hypothyroidism, thus making the person dependent on lifelong thyroid hormone supplementation. ATDs have an average remission rate of 50 percent but an excellent prognosis after 4 years without relapse.

SUBACUTE THYROIDITIS (SAI)

The term subacute thyroiditis refers to an inflammation of the thyroid gland. This is normally considered a self-limiting inflammatory disorder, which means that it will run its course usually without treatment. It is the most common cause of pain, swelling, and discomfort in the neck area. Subacute thyroiditis is thought to be initiated by a viral infection or post viral inflammatory process, often in patients with a history of an upper respiratory infection typically two to eight weeks prior to the onset of thyroiditis. The condition is believed to be triggered by an antigen created by the virus.

Individuals with SAT may also experience symptoms of hyperthyroidism (see page 80) in its early stage and hypothyroidism (see page 37) in its late stage. In most patients, SAT lasts 2 to 4 months with some people having it for one year. About two-thirds of the people with SAT will have hypothyroidism as part of the disease process.

There are many names that subacute thyroiditis may be called, such as:

- Acute simple thyroiditis
- De Quervain's thyroiditis
- Diffuse or subacute thyroiditis
- Giant cell thyroiditis
- Granulomatous thyroiditis
- Migratory creeping thyroiditis
- Noninfectious thyroiditis
- Pseudo-giant cell thyroiditis
- Pseudogranulomatous thyroiditis
- Pseudotuberculous thyroiditis
- Viral thyroiditis

SIGNS AND SYMPTOMS

The patient may experience pain in one lobe, part of a lobe, or the whole thyroid. Pain may radiate from the thyroid gland to the angle of the jaw and to the ear of the affected side. If the pain is not bilateral at first, the pain and tenderness may spread to the other side of the thyroid within days or weeks. Pain may also radiate to the anterior chest or may be centered over the thyroid. When you move your head, swallow, or cough, it may aggravate symptoms. The following are possible early signs and symptoms of SAT:

- Evidence of thyroid dysfunction
- Fatigue
- Fever

- Pharyngitis (inflammation of the back of the throat)
- Weakness

Symptoms of mild-to-moderate hyperthyroidism may occur in the early phase in many people. Pain may radiate to the jaw or the ears. Malaise, fatigue, myalgia, and arthralgia are common. A mild to moderate fever is expected, and at times a high fever of 104°F may occur. The disease process may reach its peak within 3 to 4 days and subside and disappear within a week, but more typically, onset extends over 1 to 2 weeks and continues with fluctuating intensity for 3 to 6 weeks. The thyroid gland is typically enlarged, smooth, firm, and tender to the touch. Fifty percent of individuals have symptoms of thyrotoxicosis, with nervousness, tremulousness, weight loss, heat intolerance, and tachycardia (heart racing) being the most common. Subsequently, patients often experience hypothyroidism before returning to normal. Eight to 16 percent of people with SAT have a goiter before they develop SAT. This painful condition lasts for a week to a few months, and usually demonstrates high inflammatory markers in the blood, such as very high erythrocyte sedimentation rate (ESR) and an elevated C-reactive protein (CRP) level.

CAUSES

Subacute thyroiditis has also occurred in association with outbreaks of viral infections, including the following:

- Adenovirus
- Cat-scratch fever
- Common cold
- Coxsackie virus
- Cytomegalovirus (CMV) infection
- Hepatitis A
- Influenza
- Measles
- Mononucleosis
- Mumps
- Myocarditis
- Parvovirus B19 infection
- St. Louise encephalitis
- Sars-COV-2 infection (COVID-19)

Subacute thyroiditis has occurred more frequently in association with COVID-19 than was originally considered. Two possible mechanisms of action are currently being explored. It is reasonable to hypothesize that thyrotoxicosis was caused by destructive thyroiditis. This concept is supported by the fact that thyrotoxicosis was often mild and improved spontaneously during follow-up. The close relationship between thyrotoxicosis and higher serum IL-6 (an inflammatory marker) in some studies suggests that thyroid gland inflammation may be triggered and sustained by the cytokine storm (an uncontrolled and excessive release of pro-inflammatory signaling molecules called cytokines) associated with COVID-19. An alternative theory is the possible direct action of SARS-CoV-2 on thyroid gland based on the evidence that several tissues and organs may be directly damaged by the virus during the infection. In fact, there is evidence that thyroid tissue highly expresses the angiotensin-converting enzyme 2, which is the protein used by SARS-CoV-2 for invading human cells.

SAT and SAT-like conditions have also occurred in association with other ailments, such as:

- Nonviral infections such as malaria and Q-fever
- Giant cell arteritis
- During interferon-alpha treatment for hepatitis C
- After long-term immunosuppression and lithium therapy
- Following an allogeneic bone marrow transplant

Subacute thyroiditis is uncommon but develops more frequently in women who are 40 to 50 years old than in men. SAT also more commonly occurs in North America, Japan, and Europe, which are all temperate zones. Individuals may have positive thyroid antibodies that usually decrease or normalize as the SAT resolves. Some studies have shown a T-cell mediated immunity against thyroid antigens and/or a genetic link that may play a role in the pathogenesis of SAT. Complete recovery from subacute thyroiditis is common, but recurrence after several years has been reported.

DIAGNOSIS

If an individual has had a recent viral infection, based upon any of the infections described under causes (above), the physician may request any of the following tests to be run.

Blood Tests

Inflammatory blood markers, such as sedimentation rate (sed rate), IL-6, and c-reactive protein, may be elevated. TSH is high, along with free T3 and free T4. Early on, liver enzymes may be elevated along with other blood studies. Thyroid antibodies may also be positive, in some cases a few weeks after the onset, and then decrease and disappear after the SAT is resolved. In some individuals, SAT may trigger TSH receptor antibodies to be produced, which results in TSH antibody-associated dysfunction.

Imaging Tests

Imaging tests can be administered in considering the diagnosis of SAT. These can include an ultrasound, MRI, or color Doppler ultrasound test.

Urine Test

Urinary iodine levels may be high. Due to the increased urinary excretion of iodine, it may take more than one year for the iodine stores to be replenished.

TREATMENT

In some individuals no treatment is needed for SAT. Some people will need aspirin or other anti-inflammatory medications or steroids if the case is severe. The recurrence rate is about 20 percent. Some people may develop hypothyroidism after they are treated.

Initially, other patients will become hyperthyroid and many need to be treated with beta blockers. Sodium iopodate has also been used in the treatment of hyperthyroidism related to SAT. If you have numerous recurrences, then are usually treated with thyroid medication if you are not hyperthyroid. This is to suppress TSH in order to reduce thyroid stimulation, which prolongs the inflammation. Antibiotics have not been shown to be effective. Newly, the long-term use of low-dose naltrexone (LDN) has been implemented as a wonderful therapy for this purpose. (See page 70.)

One could argue that the above approach may be not completely safe in the setting of COVID-19, since thyrotoxicosis might increase the cardiovascular risk even after short exposure to thyroid hormone excess since thyrotoxicosis may favor the development of fatal arrhythmias (irregular heart rhythms) in the presence of prolonged QT interval, a common event in COVID-19, as an effect of therapies and/or electrolyte imbalances. Moreover, the prevention and treatment of thyrotoxicosis-related heart disorders may be challenging in the setting of COVID-19, since some drugs used to counteract the negative effects of thyroid hormones on heart (for example, beta-blockers) should be administered with caution in individuals with pre-existing changes in heart rhythm.

If the subacute thyroiditis has gone on for many years, then removal of the thyroid gland may be suggested. Some people may become hypothyroid after treatment and then may require long-term therapy with thyroid medication. However, usually, the hypothyroidism that may occur is transient, so that lifelong thyroid medication is not needed.

In most cases, painless thyroiditis and subacute thyroiditis are self-limiting conditions that usually resolve spontaneously within six months. There is no role for antithyroid medications or radioactive iodine ablation in the treatment of thyroiditis. Beta blockers may be used if needed to control adrenergic symptoms. They should be used with caution in individuals with COVID-19. Pain associated with subacute thyroiditis may be relieved with a nonsteroidal anti-inflammatory drug and LDN.

OUTCOMES (PROGNOSIS)

In the majority of cases, subacute thyroiditis will need little medication, if any. However, if the condition continues for any length of time, the physician may prescribe any of the treatments related to hypo or hyperthyroidism as well as low-dose naltrexone.

SILENT OR PAINLESS THYRIODITIS (PLSAT)

Silent or painless thyroiditis is characterized by an autoimmune-mediated lymphocytic inflammation of the thyroid gland resulting in a destructive thyroiditis with release of thyroid hormone and transient thyrotoxicosis (hyperthyroidism). This is frequently followed by a hypothyroid phase before recovery of normal thyroid function. However, for some patients, the hypothyroidism is permanent. Individuals with silent thyroiditis present with symptoms of thyroiditis. Commonly, individuals with this disease alternate between experiencing symptoms of hyperthyroidism and hypothyroidism.

Although the terms silent thyroiditis and painless thyroiditis are used most commonly, many other names have been used for this disorder, including sporadic thyroiditis, destructive thyroiditis, hyperthyroiditis, spontaneously resolving lymphocytic thyroiditis, transient painless thyroiditis, painless thyroiditis with transient hyperthyroidism, painless subacute thyroiditis, occult subacute thyroiditis, atypical thyroiditis, and transient thyrotoxicosis with lymphocytic thyroiditis.

This condition is most often seen in women after delivery. It occurs in 5 to 9 percent of women in the first year, particularly in women with positive thyroid antibodies. There is a higher incidence of antimicrosomal antibodies in the postpartum form (80 percent) of the disease than in the sporadic form (50 percent). The course of the disease has four phases: thyrotoxicosis, euthyroidism (normal thyroid function), hypothyroidism, and euthyroidism. Not all four stages are present in all people. The usual course of disease is under six months for the toxic phase. The disease course is usually mild and generally you do not need treatment.

The incidence varies depending on where you may live. Silent thyroiditis is more common in Japan and uncommon in Argentina, Europe, and the east and west coasts of the United States. It is more common in the Great Lakes region and in Canada. Women up to the age of 60 and men may also be affected. Many people with silent or painless thyroiditis have a family history of the disease, including parents with postpartum thyroiditis. Exposure to iodine, such as in the form of amiodarone, lithium, interleukin 2, or interferon, may also be precipitating events. Painless or silent thyroiditis may be associated with other autoimmune diseases, such as rheumatoid arthritis, systemic sclerosis, Graves' disease, primary adrenal insufficiency, and lupus. PLSAT can also occur spontaneously. In addition, painless thyroiditis has occurred secondary to the ingestion of meat contaminated with bovine thyroid tissue. Two epidemics of thyrotoxicosis thought to reflect silent thyroiditis were found to be explained by meat contamination.

RISK FACTORS

The following are risk factors, which may cause you to be more susceptible to this disease.

Childbirth

Due to the hormonal changes in the body of a pregnant and/or postpartum female, this condition may present itself.

Genetics

Genetics seem to play a role in a person's predisposition in developing this type of thyroiditis. If a mother developed this condition after giving birth, then her daughter may develop thyroiditis after delivering a baby. However, it may require one or more triggers, as listed below, to initiate this condition. Moreover, a family history of autoimmune thyroid disease is found in 50 percent of patients with the postpartum form of thyroiditis.

Gender

Females are at higher risk to develop silent thyroiditis than males.

Infection

Painless thyroiditis may be the result of a bacterial or viral infection.

SIGNS AND SYMPTOMS

The symptoms are the same ones that you can see in thyrotoxicosis such as tachycardia, palpitations, heat intolerance, nervousness and weight loss. (See page 80.)

DIAGNOSIS

If the patient is postpartum, has an autoimmune disease, or has been exposed to iodine or medications that contain iodine, the physician my request any of the following tests to be run.

Blood Tests

Inflammatory blood markers, such as sedimentation rate (SED rate) and C-reactive protein, may be elevated. White blood cell count (WBC) is also usually high. TSH, Free T3, Free T4, reverse T3, and thyroid antibody levels will determine the state of the thyroid gland.

Imaging Tests

Imaging tests can be administered to aid in the diagnosis of silent thyroiditis. These can include an ultrasound, MRI, color Doppler ultrasound test, radioactive iodine uptake, or scan.

TREATMENT

The level of treatment is based on the severity of the condition. In some people, no treatment is required. Painless thyroiditis is a self-limiting condition that usually resolves spontaneously within six months. Anti-thyroid drugs, which inhibit the production of new T4, are not indicated in the management of patients with this form of hyperthyroidism because symptoms are caused by the release of preformed T3 and T4 and from the damaged gland. There is also no role for radioactive iodine ablation in the treatment of this form of thyroiditis. Beta blockers may be used if needed to control adrenergic symptoms. Pain associated with subacute thyroiditis may be relieved with a nonsteroidal anti-inflammatory drug.

Beta blockers were originally designed to reduce blood pressure by blocking the effects of the adrenal hormone epinephrine, also called adrenaline. It does this by slowing down the heart's beats per minute as well opening blocked vessels. This in turn reduces heart racing, palpitations, tremor, and anxiety. The effects of B-adrenergic antagonists are fast, so it is important for use early in the treatment of thyrotoxicosis. These drugs do not affect thyroid function, release, or synthesis.

In more severe cases, such as subacute thyroiditis and thyroid storm, steroids are used short term. Since this is an inflammatory disease process, the use of low-dose naltrexone (LDN) may be beneficial. See page 70 for further discussion.

OUTCOMES (PROGNOSIS)

In about half the cases, silent thyroiditis can go away on its own within one year. However, for the remainder, their condition may develop into hypothyroidism immediately or present itself years later. The hypothyroidism can become permanent, in, which case, you may be required to take a daily dose of thyroid hormone to keep your hormonal system in balance.

IODINE-INDUCED THYROTOXICOSIS (IIT)

Iodine-induced thyrotoxicosis has been recognized as early as 1821 by Coindet, who reported that goitrous individuals treated with iodine developed hyperthyroidism. The condition is now commonly called Jod-Basedow. This disease may occur in patients from endemic goiter areas, patients with multinodular goiters in non-endemic areas, individuals with Graves' disease, and in individuals without previously apparent thyroid disease. IIT has been reported due to an excess of iodine through dietary intake, also with the use of drugs or other iodine-containing compounds, contrast agents, and food components. Use of non-ionic contrast agents does not prevent the development of IIT. Thyroid hormone synthesis increases particularly in the presence of underlying thyroid disease such as multinodular goiters. In some people, the iodine-induced thyrotoxicosis effect can occur with comparatively small increases in iodine intake based on preexisting thyroid dysfunctions. When this occurs, it can lead to iodine-induced hypothyroidism symptoms (see page 37) or symptoms of thyrotoxicosis (see page 80). This condition may be temporary, or it can become permanent. There are also individuals who create their own self-induced hyperthyroidism. This condition is known as factitious hyperthyroidism and is more common than one would expect. For more information on this disorder, see page 144.

RISK FACTORS

The following are risk factors, which may cause you to be more susceptible to this disease.

Genetics

Genetics is a risk factor for individuals who have a predisposition to thyroid diseases.

Individuals With Undetected Thyroid Disease

These individuals are people that have an underlying thyroid condition and are unaware of it.

Individuals Who Are/or Have Been Treated for Either Hypo or Hyperthyroidism

In many instances, these people have been prescribed iodine supplements or antithyroid drugs to keep their thyroid hormones in balance, and any additional iodine may cause IIT. For example, euthyroid patients previously treated with antithyroid drugs for Graves' disease and nontoxic diffuse or multinodular goiters with thyroid autonomy are prone to develop iodine-induced hyperthyroidism.

Geography

Individuals with thyroid conditions living in a region where iodine consumption is very low or high may be subject to IIT.

CAUSES

Normally, this condition arises due to an existing thyroid malfunction that is undetected or being treated. Iodine-induced thyrotoxicosis is caused by an excess amount of iodine entering the body. For some the excess amount of iodine may be minimal, while for others, it may require a much larger dose for the symptoms to appear.

Antithyroid Drugs

Drugs such as interferon alpha, lithium, and amiodarone are designed to disrupt the production of thyroid hormones, destroy thyroid cells, or do both. These drugs contain iodine concentrates, which can lead to hypo or hyperthyroidism. This can then make the individual susceptible to IIT.

Radioactive Iodine Dyes

When patients undergo scans requiring a radioactive iodine dye to observe the state of their thyroid gland, they may develop IIT several weeks after administration.

Radiological contrast agents

- Diatrizoate
- Ipanoic acid
- Ipodate
- Iothalamate
- Metrizamide
- Diatrozide

Over the Counter and Prescription Drugs Containing Iodine

Drugs such as Iodochlorhydroxyquinoline, used in the treatment of prostate cancer, may bring on IIT due to its iodine content. Always ask you physician or pharmacist about the content of any drugs you may be taking.

Topical iodine preparations

- Diiodohydroxyquinolone
- Iodine tincture
- Povidone iodine
- Iodochlorohydroxyquinolone
- Iodoform gauze

Solutions

- Saturated potassium iodide (SSKI)
- Lugol solution
- Iodinated glycerol
- Echothiopate iodide
- Hydriodic acid syrup
- Calcium iodide

Drugs

- Amiodarone
- Expectorants
- Vitamins containing iodine
- Iodochlorohydroxyquinolone
- Diiodohydroxyquinolone
- Potassium iodide
- Benziodarone
- Isopropamide iodide

Antiseptics and Disinfectants

Many of the antiseptics and disinfectants used in hospitals and healthcare locations contain iodine. Tincture of iodine is commonly used on cuts and abrasions to kill bacteria.

Diet

Foods, such as shellfish, dried seaweed, cod, iodized salt, and to a lesser degree sea salt, contain iodine, which have been shown to trigger IIT. Food colors such as erythrosine iodine can also cause an elevated iodine level.

The use of iodized salt has been extensively studied. Epidemiologic studies performed in China, Turkey, and Denmark suggest that supplementation with iodized salt increases the prevalence of autoimmune thyroid disease, resulting in clinical or subclinical hypothyroidism, autoimmune hyperthyroidism, or both. In a population-based, cross-sectional study with participants exposed to excessive amounts of iodide from Brazil, the prevalence of chronic autoimmune thyroiditis was 16.9 percent, women were more commonly affected, 8 percent were hypothyroid, and 3.3 percent were hyperthyroid. The authors concluded that the excessive iodine may have increased the prevalence of autoimmune thyroid disease and hypothyroidism in this population. In Denmark, a moderately iodine-deficient country, after the introduction of iodized salt at a dose that was calculated to increase iodine intake by only 50 ug per day, an increased incidence of hyperthyroidism was found mainly in younger patients between the age of 20 and 39 years and was presumably induced by autoimmune thyroid disease. In contrast, a study on children in Morocco did not find an effect of iodine supplementation on thyroid autoimmunity.

Dietary seaweed ingestion in large amounts represents a potential source of excess iodine exposure in many parts of the world. In particular, seaweed intake is common in Asia, where it is a frequent component of the daily diet and among women during the postpartum period, who consume seaweed soup to increase the production of breastmilk. The risk of iodine-induced hyperthyroidism is also increased among individuals who consume large amounts of seaweed regularly from such sources as kelp or drinking soy milk made with kombu seaweed.

Mouthwash

Significant mild increases in serum TSH, with values remaining within the normal range, have been reported following the use of iodinated mouthwash.

Vaginal Douches

Vaginal douches have been the etiology of mild increases in TSH.

SIGNS AND SYMPTOMS

The clinical presentation includes the typical signs of thyrotoxicosis and in most patients the finding of a multinodular goiter. Other individuals may have an underlying autoimmune thyroid disease. A pre-existing thyroid disorder has been present in at least 20 percent of people. The onset of IIT may bring on many of the common issues associated with hypothyroidism and thyrotoxicosis. (See pages 37 and 80 for details.)

DIAGNOSIS

There are various tests available to determine whether you have iodine-induced thyrotoxicosis.

Physical Examination

An initial clinical diagnosis can be made based upon the medical history of the individual in conjunction with the identification of any of the possible causes of IIT listed above. When a diagnosis of IIT may be suspected, tests requiring the consumption of any substance containing iodine should be avoided. In addition, a standard examination to check blood pressure, body temperature, and heart rate will be made to determine the level of thyroid involvement.

Blood Tests

Inflammatory blood markers, such as sedimentation rate (sed rate) and c-reactive protein (CRP), may be elevated. TSH, Free T3 and Free T4, reverse T3, and thyroid antibody levels will determine the state of the thyroid gland.

TREATMENT

The treatment will depend on the cause and severity of the symptoms. It may require eliminating the underlying cause or drug therapy or both. Make sure you do not discontinue the use of any of your medications without discussing it with your healthcare provider. Spontaneous reversal to an euthyroid state may occur after a mean period of six months in about 50 percent of people. Return to normal thyroid function may be preceded by subclinical hypothyroidism.

Patient-Induced Hyperthyroidism (Factitious Hyperthyroidism) (Thyrotoxicosis Factita)

Although most cases of higher-than-normal thyroid hormone levels are caused by an overactive thyroid, this isn't always true. Sometimes, the problem occurs because the patient is taking too much thyroid hormone medication. This condition is known as factitious hyperthyroidism or thyrotoxicosis factita.

People take higher-than-prescribed doses of thyroid hormone for different reasons. In some cases, they use extra medication to lose weight, to control a menstrual disorder, to treat depression, or to treat infertility. In other cases, they have a psychiatric disorder such as Munchausen Syndrome—a mental illness in, which the person wants to be seen as having a disorder even though they have caused the symptoms themselves.

The diagnosis of factitious hyperthyroidism should be considered

Eliminating Underlying Causes

When a cause can be identified, such as a specific food or antiseptic, avoiding the cause may reduce or eliminate the symptoms. When the cause is a medication, speak to your physician regarding discontinuing its use. In some cases, there may be a severe or life-threatening reaction.

Drug Therapy

Based on the nature of the thyroid condition associated with IIT, thyroid replacement hormone is commonly prescribed if hypothyroidism is present. If the IIT has been brought about by the use of amiodarone, and the thyroid is overactive, the IIT is treated with methimazole and potassium perchlorate when identified as Type I or with prednisone when identified as Type II.

OUTCOME (PROGNOSIS)

When treated early, iodine-induced thyrotoxicosis is usually transient, and normal thyroid function should return within two to three weeks.

when laboratory tests and the physician's observations are contradictory. For instance, the individual's lab tests may reveal high levels of thyroid hormone, but they do not show the classic symptoms of Graves' disease (the most common form of hyperthyroidism), such as bulging eyes and goiter.

Symptoms of factitious hyperthyroidism normally disappear once thyroid medication dosage is lowered to the appropriate amount. The uptake of radioiodine is low and thyroglobulin levels are also very low or undetectable. The thyroid may be small. The therapy consists of appropriate dose adjustment or discontinuation of exogenous thyroid hormone.

If a psychiatric condition is responsible for the patient's excessive self-dosing, the individual will need mental health treatment to resolve the problem. Regardless of the cause, when factitious hyperthyroidism continues for a long time, it can take a heavy toll on the body. The patient should therefore be checked every two to four weeks to make sure that the thyroid levels have returned to a safe range.

Because IIT involves regaining an appropriate amount of iodine in the body in relationship to optimal thyroid hormones in the body, it is important to make sure that you have regular check-ups until the condition has been controlled or eliminated. Without an appropriate amount of thyroid hormones in the body, serious life-threatening issues can occur.

ACUTE INFECTIOUS THYROIDITIS

Because iodine is a natural antiseptic, and it is stored in high amounts in the thyroid gland, it is normally resistant to infection. In addition, its high vascularity, lymphatic drainage, the fact that hydrogen peroxide is generated within the gland as a requirement for the synthesis of thyroid hormone, and its normal encapsulated position away from external structures also makes infections less common. However, due to several existing conditions it can be infected by bacteria such as streptococcus, staphylococcus, mycobacteria, protozoa, or flatworms. Moreover, acute thyroiditis can occur in an immuno-compromised state, predisposing a person to unusual bacteria such as nocardia, salmonella, and fungi like candida, coccidioides immitis, and aspergillus.

When such an infection occurs, this condition is called acute infectious thyroiditis. It can also be referred to as chronic infectious thyroiditis, suppurative (AST), nonsuppurative, or septic thyroiditis. These types of infections are normally rare.

RISK FACTORS

The following are risk factors, which may make you more susceptible to this disease.

Abnormalities of the Piriform Sinus

This is a condition where the lower sinus cavity (called the piriform sinus) or the space connecting sinus cavities (called a fistula) becomes infected and spreads the infection to the lower portion of the neck involving the thyroid.

Compromised Immune System

Individuals with lowered immunity function may be unable to fight off a variety of infections. Any infection, such as strep bacteria, gaining a foothold in the neck area can lead to an abscess in the thyroid gland.

Other Conditions

Rarely, endocarditis (inflammation of the endocardium of the heart), tooth abscess, and fine needle aspirations may also be predisposing factors for infectious thyroiditis.

SIGNS AND SYMPTOMS

The following are symptoms you may experience when suffering from acute infectious thyroiditis:

- Fever and chills

- Local pain and tenderness in the affected lobe of the thyroid or the entire gland

- Painful swallowing and difficulty swallowing

- Pain may refer to the pharynx or ear and may be so prominent that you do not realize you have tenderness over your thyroid gland

The dominant clinical symptom is pain in the region of the thyroid gland that may subsequently enlarge and become palpably hot and tender. The person is unable to extend the neck and often sits with the neck flexed to avoid pressure on the thyroid gland. Swallowing is painful. There are usually signs of infection in structures adjacent to the thyroid, local lymphadenopathy (enlargement of lymph nodes) as well as temperature elevation and, if bacteremia (presence of bacteria in the bloodstream) occurs, chills. Gas formation with suppurative thyroiditis has been noted. Symptoms are generally more obvious in children than in adults. Adults may present with a vague slightly painful mass in the thyroid region without fever. Patients commonly present to their physician wondering if they have cancer. Suppurative thyroiditis may even spread to the chest, producing necrotizing mediastinitis (infection involving the neck and chest) and pericarditis (inflammation of the pericardium of the heart). Furthermore, infectious thyroiditis may occur more commonly in the fall and winter following upper respiratory tract infections.

DIAGNOSIS

If your physician suspects that you may have acute infectious thyroiditis a few steps will be taken to evaluate you.

Physical Examination

A standard examination to check blood pressure, body temperature, and heart rate will be made to determine the level of thyroid involvement if any. Your healthcare provider will also palpate your thyroid gland to see if it is enlarged.

Blood Tests

Inflammatory blood markers, such as sedimentation rate (sed rate) and C-reactive protein (CRP), may be elevated. TSH, Free T3 and Free T4, reverse T3, and thyroid antibody levels will determine the state of the thyroid gland. A complete blood count may be done to look for infection along with other specialized studies.

Thyroid Ultrasound

Your doctor will usually order a thyroid ultrasound if he/she suspects you have infectious thyroiditis.

Sonoelastography

Sonoelastography is an ultrasound imaging technique where low ampli-tude, low-frequency shear waves are propagated through the thyroid gland, while real-time Doppler ultrasound techniques are used to image the resulting vibration pattern. The application of sonoelastography may reveal very stiff lesions corresponding to the areas of the thyroid, which are especially painful during acute phases of the AST episode, which soften significantly as you respond to treatment.

CT Scan

A CT scan may be useful in identifying the location of the abscess. It is required only in unusual situations.

Barium Swallow

If an infectious process is identified, particularly of the left lobe of a younger individual, then a barium swallow should be performed with attention to the possibility of a fistulous tract located on the left side between the pyriform sinus and the thyroid gland. The barium swallow has very good sensitivity in detecting the presence of the fistula tracts as 89 percent to 97 percent of those examined in early and acute stages of this disease.

Blood Cultures

Blood cultures will also be drawn if your practitioner is suspicious of an infectious form of thyroiditis.

Fine Needle Aspiration (FNA)

A fine needle aspiration is taken. The skin above the node is numbed and a thin needle is inserted into the area to remove cells for review. These samples are then sent to a laboratory where a pathologist examines them under a microscope to determine the exact source of the infection. The pathologist writes up a report on his findings and sends back the report to the ordering doctor.

TREATMENT

Based on the type of infection found, treatments usually include antibiotics or antifungal agents. Microscopic examination and appropriate staining of a fine needle aspiration often aid the diagnosis and choice of antibiotic therapy. The choice of therapy will also depend on the immune status of the patient. Systemic antibiotics are required for severe infections. Candida albicans thyroiditis may be treated with appropriate doses of amphotericin B and fluconazole. Successful antifungal combination therapy and a surgical approach for Aspergillus spp-associated AST have been reported. Nonsteroidal anti-inflammatory drugs (NSAIDs) are used to control severe neck pain and inflammation. The newest therapy to control inflammation is low-dose naltrexone (LDN). (See the section on LDN on page 70) Surgical intervention, like abscess drainage, can be done if clinically indicated. The disease may occasionally prove fatal, particularly if the patient does not seek healthcare early in the disease course. In some people with thyroiditis, the destruction may be sufficiently severe that permanent hypothyroidism results. Therefore, individuals with diffuse thyroiditis should have follow-up thyroid function studies performed to determine the need for thyroid hormone replacement.

OUTCOME (PROGNOSIS)

With the appropriate treatment, this condition is usually resolved.

HYPERTHYROIDISM AND GESTATIONAL TROPHOBLASTIC DISORDERS

PREGNANCY AND HYPERTHYROIDISM

Human chorionic gonadotropin (hCG) is a hormone that is produced in a pregnant woman. In part, hCG is responsible for nausea during the first trimester of pregnancy. During pregnancy, transient gestational thyrotoxicosis may be due to stimulation of the TSH receptor by high levels of hCG since it has intrinsic TSH-like activity. In 10 to 20 percent of normal pregnancies the hCG-induced hyperthyroidism goes undetected (subclinical). Actual hCG-induced hyperthyroidism occurs in about 1.4 percent of pregnant women where they have symptoms of hyperthyroidism. With multiple births, the hCG levels are even higher. During the early stages of pregnancy, approximately 5 percent of woman experience nausea and vomiting along with weight loss. This is called hyperemesis gravidarum syndrome and is due to a woman's higher levels of hCG. The degree of biochemical hyperthyroidism and hCG concentration correlate directly with the severity of vomiting. Additionally, gestational transient thyrotoxicosis can also occur due to a gene mutation, which makes the body hypersensitive to hCG.

RISK FACTORS

The following are risk factors, which may make you more susceptible to this disease.

Pregnancy

Pregnancy brings on several hormonal changes in a woman's body. There is a rapid rise in levels of estrogen and progesterone as well as hCG. hCG and TSH share the common glycoprotein alpha subunit and the beta subunit. At high doses, hCG cross-reacts with the TSH receptor, and this stimulation can lead to an increase in secretion of T4 and T3, with subsequent suppression of TSH secretion. Therefore, the thyroid gland of normal pregnant women may be stimulated by hCG to secrete slightly excessive quantities of T4 and induce a slight suppression of TSH, but it only induces overt hyperthyroidism in some pregnant women.

Genetics

Genetics is a risk factor for pregnant women who have a predisposition to thyroid disease.

Preexisting Thyroid Disease

There may be several thyroid problems such as Graves' disease, an autoimmune-based disorder of the thyroid, which may have gone undetected prior to the pregnancy.

SIGNS AND SYMPTOMS

While some hCG-related symptoms are common during pregnancy, should these symptoms become excessive, you should contact your physician and consider the possibility of checking your thyroid hormone levels. For a complete list of hyperthyroid symptoms, see page 80.

- Diarrhea
- Enlarged thyroid gland
- Excessive sweating
- Fast heartbeat (tachycardia)
- Mood changes

- Nausea
- Trouble sleeping
- Vomiting
- Weight loss or gaining weight too slowly

DIAGNOSIS

If your physician suspects that you may have developed hyperthyroidism, various steps will be taken.

Physical Examination

A standard examination to check blood pressure, body temperature, and heart rate will be made to determine the level of thyroid involvement, if any, along with the usual examination that occurs at a prenatal visit.

Blood Tests

Results are normally based on high levels of free T3 and free T4 levels and low levels of TSH to determine the potential of hyperthyroidism. hCG levels are also measured on a regular basis.

Urine Test

Analyzing the thyroid hormone levels in the urine may be used as an adjunct to a blood test to indicate the status of the thyroid gland.

TREATMENT

With moderate hCG levels, there are usually no treatments necessary. Normally, this type of condition is termed "self-limiting," since it will resolve itself after childbirth. When the symptoms are more severe, treatment is important, but may be limited owing to the safety of the baby. Treatments may include the following:

Anti-thyroid drugs. Of the three thionamide drugs, propylthiouracil (PTU) is preferred during first trimester of pregnancy. This drug is used to stop the production of TSH with fewer side effects.

Beta-blockers. These medications may be used to slow the mother's heart rate down and reduce tremors.

OUTCOME (PROGNOSIS)

For the majority of pregnant women, "morning sickness" is part of the ritual of having a baby. Its underlying cause is of little concern since it clears up by the later stages of pregnancy. However, for some women, the symptoms may be much more severe and should be treated or at the very least, monitored by a physician. If left untreated, hyperthyroidism can have serious consequences to both mother and child.

HYDATIDIFORM MOLES

Hydatidiform moles can lead to high hCG levels and thyrotoxicosis. A molar pregnancy (hydatidiform mole) is when a mass of tissue grows inside your uterus that will not develop into a baby. It is the result of abnormal conception. It is a is a subcategory of diseases under gestational trophoblastic disease (GTD), which originates from the placenta and can metastasize. It is unique because the tumor originates from gestational tissue rather than from maternal tissue. Hydatidiform mole is categorized as a complete or partial mole and is usually considered the noninvasive form of gestational trophoblastic disease. Although hydatidiform moles are usually considered benign, they are considered premalignant and do have the potential to become malignant and invasive.

RISK FACTORS

The following are risk factors for hydatidiform moles.

Genetics

Recurrent hydatidiform moles are linked to an autosomal recessive disease with biparental karyotype (BiCHM), termed as familial recurrent hydatidiform moles. Thereby, in women with recurrent pregnancy loss, mutations in NLRP7 gene (OMIM 609661) and less frequently in KHDC3L gene (OMIM 611687) could be detected.

Previous Molar Pregnancy

The risk for molar pregnancy is increased by 1 percent to 2 percent after one, and by 15 to 20 percent after two prior molar pregnancies.

Age

The occurrence of a molar pregnancy strongly correlates with maternal age especially for women younger than 16 years and even more pronounced for those above 45 years.

SIGNS AND SYMPTOMS

Most women with hydatidiform moles present with uterine bleeding in the first half of pregnancy. The size of the uterus is large for the duration of gestation. Many women with molar pregnancies have nausea and vomiting, and some have pregnancy-induced hypertension or (pre)-eclampsia. Anemia, uterine enlargement, and respiratory distress may also appear. The signs and symptoms of thyrotoxicosis are present in some women, but they may be obscured by toxemic signs. The characteristic features belonging to Graves' disease are usually missing. Thyrotoxicosis is usually not severe because of a relatively short duration.

DIAGNOSIS

Since the definitive diagnosis cannot be obtained by histology in most cases, persistent or recurrent disease is diagnosed by elevated or persistent serum levels of hCG. If symptoms of hyperthyroidism are present, then your healthcare provider will also measure thyroid studies.

Physical Examination

A standard examination to check blood pressure, body temperature, and heart rate will be made to determine the level of thyroid involvement.

Blood Tests

Results are normally based on high levels of T3 and Free T4 levels and low levels of TSH to determine the potential of hyperthyroidism. Measurement of serum hCG concentrations is needed for the diagnosis of moles, and hCG serves as a sensitive and specific tumor marker during therapy and surveillance. In women, hCG concentrations are significantly higher than those found during normal pregnancies.

Ultrasound

Ultrasonography of the uterus shows an enlarged uterus. In addition, the classic indicators for GTD are the ultrasonographic display of a characteristic "snowstorm" pattern and theca lutein ovarian cysts.

TREATMENT

Hydatidiform moles are treated by suction dilation and curettage performed under ultrasonographic vision to avoid perforation of the uterus. In cases of life-threatening hemorrhage, hysterectomy is recommended. Besides a variety of different protocols for follow-up, the recommendation of the International Federation of Gynecology and Obstetrics (FIGO) has been generally accepted. Women with a partial hydatidiform mole should be followed up by weekly hCG controls to record a normal level of hCG in two consecutive measurements, followed by monthly check-ups for the next 3 to 6 months. Complete hydatidiform moles require monthly check-ups for an entire year. Additionally, patients should be instructed to use contraception for a period of least one year to enable conclusive follow-up processes. To avoid perforation of the uterus, intrauterine devices (IUDs) should not be used for contraception. In addition, if you have had a histology of a molar pregnancy, your doctor will check hCG levels 6 and 10 weeks after each subsequent pregnancy to detect a possible relapse of previous molar disease.

OUTCOMES (PROGNOSIS)

In individuals with hydatidiform moles, serum free T4, free T3, TSH, and hCG levels normalize rapidly after removal of the mole. In patients with low risk choriocarcinomas, the success rate is close to 100 percent.

CHORIOCARCINOMA

There are two forms of choriocarcinoma, gestational and non-gestational. The gestational form arises following a hydatidiform mole, normal pregnancy, or most commonly, spontaneous abortion, while non-gestational choriocarcinoma arises from pluripotent germ cells.

Gestational choriocarcinoma is a rare tumor with varied incidence worldwide. In Europe and North America, about 1 in 40,000 pregnant patients and 1 in 40 patients with hydatidiform moles will develop choriocarcinoma. In Southeast Asia and Japan, 9.2 in 40,000 pregnant women and 3.3 in 40 patients with hydatidiform moles will subsequently develop choriocarcinoma.

Non-gestational choriocarcinomas form in males or females. These tumors can be found in areas other than the uterus. They may develop in the ovaries, vagina, testicles, chest, or abdomen. In these cases, choriocarcinoma is usually mixed with other types of cancer, forming a type of cancer called a mixed germ cell tumor. Choriocarcinoma in males, usually occur between the ages of 20 to 30. Less than 1 percent of testicular tumors are pure choriocarcinoma. Mixed germ cell tumors occur much more frequently in the testicle, with choriocarcinoma as a component in 15 percent of these tumors.

Choriocarcinoma is an aggressive, highly malignant tumor in both forms.

RISK FACTORS

The following are risk factors for gestational choriocarcinomas.

Pregnancy

It is of particular importance that choriocarcinomas can occur after any kind of pregnancy. However, it is mainly diagnosed after a hydatidiform mole.

Other Risk Factors

There is a slight risk of developing gestational choriocarcinoma if you:

- Are currently pregnant
- Were recently pregnant
- Had an abortion
- Had a miscarriage

- Long-term use of oral contraceptives
- Genetic: overexpression of p53 and MDM2
- Blood type A
- Had an ectopic pregnancy (fertilized egg is implanted outside the uterus)
- Had a vaginal or other genital tumor

SIGNS AND SYMPTOMS

Signs and symptoms vary between women and men.

- For women, besides vaginal bleeding and dysmenorrhea, further non-specific symptoms such as nausea or hemoptysis (coughing up blood from your lungs) may only be seen after the tumor has spread to different organs. Women may also present with hyperthyroidism.

- In men, they may develop gynecomastia (breast enlargement) and/or hyperthyroidism. Males may also have symptoms of metastatic disease such as hemoptysis, but the liver, GI tract, and brain are also frequently involved.

DIAGNOSIS

Since choriocarcinomas can occur even years after any pregnancy, the diagnosis is challenging under these circumstances. The diagnosis in males is commonly made late, as well, when metastasis has already occurred.

Physical Examination

A standard examination to check blood pressure, body temperature, and heart rate will be made to determine the level of thyroid involvement, if any. A pelvic examination will also be performed in female patients. A urological evaluation will be conducted on males. In males who have developed choriocarcinoma, the testicular anatomy is usually very small or even regressed, leaving only metastatic disease and cells.

Blood Tests

Serum test results are normally based on high levels of free T3 and free T4 levels and low levels of TSH to determine the potential of hyperthyroidism. Measurement of serum hCG concentrations is needed for the diagnosis of choriocarcinomas, and hCG serves as a sensitive and specific tumor marker during therapy and surveillance. In women, hCG concentrations are significantly higher than those found during normal pregnancies.

Ultrasound

Women with choriocarcinomas present within one year after conception. The tumor may be confined to the uterus, more frequently it is metastatic to multiple organs such as the liver and lungs, among others. In men, choriocarcinomas of the testes is often widely metastatic at initial presentation. Gynecomastia is a common finding.

TREATMENT

When it comes to treatment, choriocarcinomas can be divided into two groups: 1) a low-risk group treated by monotherapy, most often with methotrexate or actinomycin D and 2) a high-risk group treated with polychemotherapy (etoposide, methotrexate, actinomycin D, cyclophosphamide, vincristine) with a response of about 86 percent. Longitudinal measurement of hCG as a specific and sensitive tumor marker is key for long-term surveillance. Placental-site trophoblastic tumors, a rare form of gestational trophoblastic disease that does not secrete hCG, requires stage-adapted management with surgery, or surgery in combination with chemotherapy. Non-gestational choriocarcinomas are now also treated successfully with chemotherapy.

OUTCOMES (PROGNOSIS)

Gestational choriocarcinoma and non-gestational choriocarcinoma have different prognoses, with non-gestational choriocarcinoma having a much worse prognosis. Low-risk gestational choriocarcinoma has almost 100 percent survival in women treated with chemotherapy, and high-risk gestational choriocarcinoma patients have 91 percent to 93 percent survival when utilizing multi-agent chemotherapy with or without radiation and surgery. In patients that are not responding to chemotherapy, the 5-year survival rate is about 43 percent. In men with mixed germ cell tumors, increasing amounts of choriocarcinoma suggest a worse prognosis. The good news is that novel chemotherapeutic agents are currently being used on a regular basis to improve outcomes. In addition, the use of low-dose naltrexone as part of the therapy in some oncology centers has been shown to be beneficial. See page 70 for more information on LDN.

STRUMA OVARII

Struma ovarii is a variant of dermoid tumors of the ovary in, which thyroid tissue components are the major constituent. Thyroid tissue is observed not uncommonly in 5 to 15 percent of dermoid tumors, but to be called a struma ovarii tumor the thyroid proportion must comprise more than 50 percent of the overall tissue. It rarely causes hyperthyroidism. Most individuals with struma ovarii clinically and biochemically have normal thyroid function.

Struma ovarii of the ovary is a relatively rare tumor, which comprises 1 percent of all ovarian tumors and 2.7 percent of all dermoid tumors. It forms less than 1 percent of all ovarian tumors and 2 percent to 4 percent of all ovarian teratomas; 5 to 10 percent are bilateral (involving both sides); and 5 to 10 percent are malignant (cancerous). Thyrotoxicosis occurs in about 8 percent of affected patients.

RISK FACTORS

The two known risk factors are age (between 40 to 60 years old) and post-menopausal status.

SIGNS AND SYMPTOMS

The clinical presentation may include the findings of an abdominal mass, ascites (the accumulation of fluid in the peritoneal cavity causing abdominal swelling), pelvic pain, abnormal vaginal bleeding, hydrothorax (fluid in the pleural cavity), and, rarely, pseudo-Meigs syndrome with pleural effusions (the build-up of excess fluid between the layers of the pleura outside of the lungs). A subset of women present with subclinical or overt thyrotoxicosis. Goiter is only present in patients with associated thyroid disease. Furthermore, the coexistence of Graves' disease and struma ovarii has been reported.

DIAGNOSIS

Pre-operatively struma ovarii are difficult to diagnosis.

Physical Examination

A standard examination to check blood pressure, body temperature, and heart rate will be made to determine the level of thyroid involvement if any. A pelvic examination will also be performed.

Imaging Tests: Ovaries and Thyroid

Pre-operative radiologic imaging studies such as ultrasonography were able to diagnose struma ovarii in only 11.8 percent of patients in one study. Other pre-operative diagnoses, which were later confirmed to be struma ovarii were dermoid tumors (a bizarre tumor, usually benign, in the ovary that typically contains a diversity of tissues including hair, teeth, bone, thyroid, etc.), benign cysts, and endometriomas (cysts that form on the ovaries when endometrial tissue grows on the ovaries). In other words, the diagnosis is not always clear before surgery because it is difficult to distinguish between struma ovarii and dermoid cysts on the basis of ultrasound. Doppler flow may aid in the pre-operative diagnosis. Blood flow signals, detected from the center of the echoic lesion, and low resistance to flow may be common in individuals with struma ovarii. Cross-sectional imaging with computed tomography (CT) or magnetic resonance imaging (MRI) will demonstrate unilateral or bilateral (both sides) ovarian masses.

A radioactive iodine uptake test (RAIU) is typically performed with a thyroid scan to assist in determining thyroid health and function. This test helps to see how much radioactive iodine your thyroid has absorbed over a certain time period, usually 6 or 24 hours after taking radioactive iodine. Radioiodine uptake will reveal uptake in the pelvis, while the uptake in the thyroid is diminished or absent. Furthermore, an ultrasound of the thyroid gland may be helpful. Rarely, women with struma ovarii and hyperthyroidism also have a goiter.

Blood Work

In individuals with thyrotoxicosis, TSH is suppressed and T3 and T4 levels are elevated. Thyroglobulin is secreted by benign and malignant ovarian strumae.

Moreover, CA125 may be elevated. This widely accepted tumor marker of ovarian cancers, CA-125, is found to be increased in 80 percent of epithelial ovarian carcinomas. This marker is also elevated in other tumorous lesions of the endometrium (mucous membrane lining the uterus), intestines, breasts, and lungs, as well as in non-malignant related gynecologic conditions, thus indicating that there is a limit to the clinical application of CA-125 as a tumor marker for malignant ovarian neoplasms.

TREATMENT

Treatment consists of surgical removal of the teratoma via unilateral or bilateral open or laparoscopic oophorectomy (surgical procedure to remove one or both of the ovaries) as the primary therapy. The occurrence of ascites in patients with struma ovarii has been observed to vary, ranging from 17 percent to 33.3 percent, according to several authors. The precise mechanisms of the formation of ascites in struma ovarii patients are unclear, but it has been suggested that ascites, if present, usually regresses spontaneously after surgical removal of struma ovarii. For individuals with multiple metastatic lesion or those who do absorb radioiodine poorly, external beam radiation has been proposed. For advanced stage disease (cancer) the surgical protocol is the same as for epithelial ovarian cancers. A recent proposal has been put forward in, which surgical resection of tumor is accompanied by radioiodine therapy, but this has not been further substantiated.

Thyrotoxic women are treated with antithyroid drugs and, if needed, with beta-blockers prior to surgery. In non-cancerous cases, thyroid laboratory findings usually normalize after surgery. In the case of malignant lesions of the thyroid, the patient should undergo thyroidectomy followed by treatment with 1-131 iodine. The subsequent surveillance for residual or recurrent thyroid cancer does not differ from primary thyroid carcinomas. (See Chapter 18 on page 297.)

OUTCOMES (PROGNOSIS)

Cases of malignant struma ovarii may need adjuvant treatment, but recurrence is uncommon. Also, it should be remembered that ovarian tumors can cause hyperthyroidism. Controlling the thyroid hormone level preoperatively by using antithyroid drugs, and performing minimally invasive laparoscopic surgery, is considered useful for preventing thyroid storm.

DRUG-ASSOCIATED HYPERTHYROIDISM

Amiodarone is an antiarrhythmic medication (drug used to treat abnormal heart rates or rhythms) that is 37 percent iodine by weight and has a half-life of approximately 100 days. Amiodarone-induced thyroid dysfunction is a particular concern in individuals with underlying thyroid disease and is estimated to induce thyroid dysfunction in 15 percent to 20 percent of people who take this medication. Furthermore, amiodarone-induced hypothyroidism is more common in iodine-sufficient areas of the world, whereas amiodarone-induced hyperthyroidism is seen more frequently in iodine-deficient regions. Amiodarone-induced thyrotoxicosis has been divided into types 1 and type 2.

- Type 1 amiodarone-induced thyrotoxicosis is a form of iodine-induced thyrotoxicosis that is more prevalent among individuals with pre-existing thyroid disease living in regions of low iodine intake and occurs secondary to the Jod–Basedow phenomenon (hyperthyroidism following administration of iodine or iodide or taking a medication containing iodine). It is treated with a combination of antithyroid medications, beta-blockade, and, if available, perchlorate, to decrease the entrance of iodine into the thyroid.

- Type 2 amiodarone-induced thyrotoxicosis is a destructive thyroiditis in, which thyrotoxicosis results from thyroid hormone release from the gland. It usually occurs in people with no history of thyroid disease. The prevalence of type 2 in iodine-deficient regions is estimated to be 5 to 10 percent and occurs in a male-to-female ratio of 3:1. Treatment is primarily steroids.

The ability to distinguish between the two types of amiodarone-induced thyrotoxicosis is often challenging, and a mixed presentation may occur in some individuals. Amiodarone should not be discontinued unless it can be stopped safely, without triggering heart complications.

Hyperthyroidism associated with use of other medications (e.g., lithium, interferon alfa, tyrosine kinase inhibitors, and highly active antiretroviral therapy) is usually self-limiting. Your physician will determine whether the medication may be discontinued safely or replaced with a different medication.

TSH-SECRETING ADENOMAS (TSHomas)

TSH-secreting adenomas (TSHomas) account for less than 2 percent of all pituitary adenomas and are a rare cause of thyrotoxicosis. TSHomas and thyroid hormone resistance form the two syndromes of "inappropriate TSH secretion," defined by normal or elevated TSH levels in combination with increased free T4 and free T3 levels. Individuals with TSHomas present with signs and symptoms of hyperthyroidism and an enlarged thyroid. In patients with resistance to thyroid hormone, the phenotype is more complex as some tissues are resistant to the action of the elevated peripheral hormones and thus hypothyroid, whereas other tissues can be excessively stimulated. The physiological negative feedback normally exerted by thyroid hormones is not operating in both conditions. TSHomas secrete TSH in an autonomous fashion, in resistance to thyroid hormone, the thyrotropes (endocrine cells in the anterior pituitary, which produce TSH) are resistant to the high levels of thyroid hormone.

RISK FACTORS

The molecular mechanisms leading to the formation of TSHomas remain unknown. TSHomas have been shown to be monoclonal by X-inactivation analyses suggesting that they arise from a single cell harboring one or several mutations in genes controlling proliferation (rapid increase in numbers) and perhaps function. Most patients are older, but TSHomas have also been documented in children.

SIGNS AND SYMPTOMS

Individuals with a TSHoma typically present with signs of hyperthyroidism, particularly signs that are related to pressure, such as vision loss and headaches. The majority of cases of TSHoma present with visual symptoms.

DIAGNOSIS

Physical Examination

A standard examination to check blood pressure, body temperature, and heart rate will be made to determine the level of thyroid involvement.

Blood Work

In individuals with thyrotoxicosis, TSH is suppressed and T3 and T4 levels are elevated. Some clinicians measure the glycoprotein alpha subunit as a marker to distinguish between TSHomas and resistance to thyroid hormone. Other pituitary hormones, prolactin, FSH, and LH should also be measured. Thyrotropin-releasing hormone (TRH) is a hormone produced by neurons in the hypothalamus that stimulate the release of TSH and prolactin from the pituitary. TRH is also commonly measured.

Imaging Tests

Magnetic resonance imaging (MRI) of the pituitary will reveal a pituitary adenoma in individuals with TSHomas.

TREATMENT

Complete resection may not be possible because these tumors can invade the sinus cavernosus and other adjacent structures. Prior to surgery, hyperthyroidism should be controlled with thionamides and beta-blockers. In patients with residual tumor tissue and persistent secretion of TSH, both gamma knife radiotherapy and medical therapies can be considered. Drug therapies include the use of somatostatin analogues, such as octreotide and lanreotide. TSHomas express somatostatin receptors and therefore somatostatin analogues are highly effective in reducing TSH secretion by neoplastic thyrotropes. If tolerated, somatostatin analogues are effective in reducing TSH secretion in more than 90 percent of individuals with consequent normalization of thyroid hormone levels and restoration of the euthyroid state. Tumor shrinkage does occur in all people.

OUTCOMES (PROGNOSIS)

In the case of a surgical cure, the postoperative TSH is undetectable and may remain low for weeks or months, causing central hypothyroidism. Permanent central hypothyroidism may also occur due to the mass effect exerted by the tumor or after radiotherapy. Thus, short-term or long-term thyroid hormone replacement may be necessary. Long-term evaluation of all pituitary hormones is important, particularly in individuals who underwent radiotherapy, in order to recognize and treat anterior pituitary deficiencies in a timely manner.

THYROID HORMONE RESISTANCE

Thyroid hormone resistance (THR) is a rare syndrome of reduced end organ sensitivity. THR is defined by elevated circulating levels of free thyroid hormones due to reduced target tissue responsiveness and normal, or elevated, levels of TSH. As discussed above, it is one of the two conditions that are part of "inappropriate TSH secretion." It is an inherited condition that occurs in 1 of 40,000 live births characterized by a reduced responsiveness of target tissues to thyroid hormone due to mutations on the thyroid hormone receptor.

RISK FACTORS

Thyroid hormone resistance is differentiated from thyroid stimulating hormone (TSH) secreting pituitary adenoma by history of thyroid hormone resistance in the family. The most well-known cause of the syndrome are mutations of the β (beta) form (THRB gene) of the thyroid hormone receptor, of, which over 100 different mutations have been documented. Mutations in MCT8 and SECISBP2 have also been associated with this condition.

SIGNS AND SYMPTOMS

Most individuals present with signs of hyperthyroidism. The most common symptoms are goiter and tachycardia (heart racing). It should also be noted that the elevation of free thyroid hormone levels does not always result in thyrotoxicosis in all tissues. Thyroid hormone resistance has also been linked to some cases of attention deficit hyperactivity disorder (ADHD), although the majority of people with that diagnosis have no thyroid problems. Moreover, some people complain of "brain fog." An association with depression has also been proposed.

DIAGNOSIS

The diagnosis involves identifying a mutation of the thyroid receptor, which is present in approximately 85 percent of cases.

Physical Examination

A standard examination to check blood pressure, body temperature, and heart rate will be made to determine the level of thyroid involvement if any. The patient commonly presents with a goiter on physical examination.

Blood Work

Patients with thyroid hormone resistance usually have elevated thyroid hormones and a normal or elevated thyroid-stimulating hormone level. The person's metabolic state may appear normal or include signs of hypothyroidism or hyperthyroidism. In patients with resistance to thyroid hormones, the characteristics are complex, as some tissues are resistant to the action of the elevated peripheral hormones and thus hypothyroid, whereas other tissues can be excessively stimulated. The physiological negative feedback normally exerted by thyroid hormones is not operating.

Imaging Tests

Patients with thyroid hormone resistance typically present with a goiter. Consequently, an ultrasound of the thyroid is usually performed. Ultrasonography uses sound waves to create a computerized image of tissues in your neck. The technician uses a wand-like device (transducer) over your neck to do the test. This imaging technique can reveal the size of your thyroid gland and detect nodules.

TREATMENT

No specific treatment is often required for thyroid hormone resistance; patients with features of hypothyroidism are treated with thyroid replacement. Beta blockers, like metoprolol, are sometimes used to help suppress symptoms of hyperthyroidism. The goiter is usually of little consequence. However, in the occasion of larger symptomatic goiter, a surgical approach is usually ineffective, as the goiter tends to reoccur. Therefore, it is logical to target TSH suppression to inhibit thyroid gland growth.

Thyroid nodules are quite prevalent in the general population and thus may occasionally co-exist with thyroid resistance. Although the majority of thyroid nodules are benign and do not require surgical management, there are few reported cases of papillary thyroid carcinoma in people with resistance to thyroid hormone. In these cases, thyroidectomy and radioactive iodine ablation to prevent disease recurrence result in lifelong thyroid hormone replacement therapy and persistently high serum TSH. Alternative options to consider include 3,3,5-triiodothyroacetic acid

(TRIAC), a thyroid hormone analogue with thyromimetic effects on pituitary and liver tissue that may be used to suppress TSH, and combination of levothyroxine (T4) with beta-blocker to alleviate tachycardia (heart racing) along with calcium and vitamin D supplementation to prevent bone loss acceleration.

Attention deficit disorder (ADHD), reported in 48 percent to 83 percent of individuals with thyroid resistance and is treated using conventional drugs. When such medications are ineffective, treatment with T3 was found beneficial in reducing impulsivity in 5 of 8 and hyperactivity in 4 of 7 individuals with resistance to thyroid hormone and ADHD but not in individuals with ADHD only. Every other day T3 therapy was also effective to improve insomnia and hyperactivity in a young child with severe thyroid resistance phenotype intolerant to daily levothyroxine (T4) therapy.

OUTCOMES (PROGNOSIS)

Thyroid hormone resistance is an autosomal dominant or recessive inherited disease with different clinical manifestations and generally does not require treatment. In cases with obvious thyrotoxicosis, TRIAC is effective, and beta-blocker treatment may be considered for people with obvious tachycardia. For individuals with hypothyroidism, thyroid hormone replacement can be considered. There are no guidelines or expert consensus on the treatment of thyroid resistance accompanied by other diseases, and thus further research is needed. The syndrome should be suspected in patients with increased serum thyroid level, accompanied by a normal or elevated TSH concentration. The affected patients require individualized management.

CONCLUSION

While some of the thyroid-related disorders discussed in this chapter are relatively rare, to an individual who suffers from one of these conditions being rare means very little. What is important is identifying the problem, understanding what it is, and then knowing what your options are. Don't be afraid to ask your physician questions and act as your own advocate. As you will see in the upcoming chapters, your thyroid gland has a great deal to do with many aspects of your well-being.

7

Thyroid Hormones and Your Memory

While you have seen how important thyroid hormones are to our overall metabolism, what you may not be aware of is the important role they play in keeping our brain functioning properly. As the center of our thought process, nervous system, and sensory capabilities, any chemical imbalances in this complex organ can have a significant impact in your daily lives. As you will see, such an impact can stem directly from improper thyroid hormone production—specifically on your ability to remember and focus.

Since thyroid hormones regulate every cell and organ of the body, it is not surprising that optimal thyroid hormone function is essential to the brain and its many activities, including the ability to form and preserve memory. Studies have shown that challenges with thyroid function—even at a subclinical (undetected) level when no obvious symptoms are present—can affect the brain in many ways.

This chapter first explores how thyroid hormone imbalances are known to influence a range of mental (cognitive) processes, including the acquisition of information, the ability to focus, the capacity to solve problems, and, of course, memory. It then looks at several specific forms of thyroid dysfunction, how they impact the brain, and how they can be treated.

AN OVERVIEW OF THE EFFECT OF THYROID PROBLEMS ON COGNITIVE FUNCTION AND MEMORY

Studies in both animals and humans have provided abundant evidence that thyroid hormone problems, whether they involve the production of too little thyroid hormone or too much thyroid hormone, can affect brain function in several ways since thyroid hormones play a role in brain areas that are crucial for our memory and cognitive skills. They can impair the growth of the neurons that allow the transmission of brain messages, and they can influence the chemical substances vital to the transmission of these messages. Likewise, thyroid hormones affect other hormones, such as pregnenolone (your hormone of memory), estrogen, progesterone, testosterone, DHEA, cortisol, and insulin, which also have a direct effect on memory, and they can furthermore directly affect the portion of the brain responsible for memory.

Hypothyroidism, including hypothyroidism related to Hashimoto's thyroiditis, (see Chapters 2 and 3) have been found to impair neurogenesis, the growth and development of the neurons. Since neurons are the specialized cells that carry messages within the human brain, problems with neurogenesis can lead to reduced cognitive function.

The portion of the brain called the hippocampus is involved in forming, storing, and processing memory. As you might suspect, any condition that adversely affects this important structure also harms cognitive abilities. There are two hippocampus regions; one located on the left side of the brain, and the other on the right. These areas play an important role in storing short-term and long-term memory as well as giving you a sense of spatial navigation. In Alzheimer's disease, the hippocampus is one of the first areas of the brain to suffer damage resulting in memory loss or disorientation. When adult-onset hypothyroidism hampers hippocampal neurogenesis—the development of neurons within the hippocampus—both learning and memory are affected. Studies on animals have suggested that this impairment in memory may be related to damage to long-term potentiation (LTP), which is the strengthening of connections between neurons that supports signal transmission and enables the formation of memories. Fortunately, it has been found that replacement of T4—thyroxine, one of the thyroid hormones—can restore LTP and thus improve both learning and memory.

Several studies have highlighted the importance of T4 to cognitive function. One study showed that when laboratory animals received T4 replacement, their learning ability for spatial tasks was enhanced. It is believed that the animals' improved learning was related to a healthier cholinergic system—the system that helps govern the learning process.

Moreover, studies have also demonstrated that levels of thyroid-stimulating hormone (TSH), which regulates the production of both T4 and

T3 (triiodothyronine), are related to measures of attention. It also shows low levels of TSH may predict vascular dementia, a form of dementia caused by impaired blood supply to the brain. To be specific, hypothyroidism is associated with increased risk of dementia. This association is influenced by both comorbidity (the presence of two or more medical conditions) and age. One trial revealed that for every six months of elevated TSH, it increased the risk of dementia by 12 percent, suggesting that the length of hypothyroidism also influences the risk of memory loss.

T4 is not the only thyroid hormone that is involved in cognitive function. Normally, the thyroid hormones that are active in the brain have receptors that aid in carrying out these crucial activities. The thyroid hormone T3 has two receptors: alpha and beta, which are paramount for focus and memory. Therefore, having enough T3 is important. In fact, both low *and* high levels of T3 have been found to result in severe cognitive problems. As you have seen previously, hypothyroidism is associated with cognitive changes. Graves' hyperthyroid patients—who have increased levels of T3—tend to also experience problems with memory, attention, and complex problem solving. (See page 174 of this chapter for more about Graves' disease and cognition.) Moreover, optimal levels of T3 are vital for focus and memory as are optimal levels of TSH. One study showed that for every 6 months of decreased TSH was associated with increased risk of dementia by 16 percent, compared with individuals with normal TSH. Therefore, the data supports early diagnosis and intervention in patients with hyperthyroidism.

Thyroid function has also been found to affect the function of neurotransmitters, the chemicals that transmit signals from one neuron to another neuron, as well as the function of neuromodulators, the chemicals that stimulate neuron function. See the next chapter for a longer explanation of neurotransmitter function in the body and its relationship to thyroid function. As research continues, more will be learned about the many ways in, which thyroid hormones influence memory and other cognitive abilities. At this point, studies have shown that optimal levels of thyroid hormones are vital for normal brain function.

FORMS OF THYROID DYSFUNCTION THAT AFFECT BRAIN FUNCTION

There are four common types of thyroid dysfunction that can affect cognition: overt hypothyroidism, subclinical hypothyroidism, overt hyperthyroidism, and subclinical hyperthyroidism. The remainder of this chapter examines these disorders and their relationship to focus and memory. Finally, this chapter looks at a rare form of thyroid dysfunction called Hashimoto's encephalopathy, which can have a profound effect on cognitive function.

OVERT HYPOTHYROIDISM

Overt hypothyroidism is hypothyroidism (low thyroid function) that can be measured by laboratory tests and manifests itself in obvious symptoms. It occurs when the thyroid gland is underactive and does not produce enough thyroid hormones.

When the production of the thyroid hormones slows down, this leads to impairments in cholinergic system and hypothalamus, and consequently, you can experience these effects via symptoms such as brain fog. Two recent trials revealed that symptoms of hypothyroidism-associated brain fog vary among patients but commonly include fatigue, depressed mood, and cognitive difficulties in the areas of memory and executive function. In addition, scientists have observed that hypothyroidism can lead to impaired nerve cell generation in the hippocampus (the brain's memory center), behavioral alterations, and cognitive deficits. Moreover, thyroid hormones may serve to support long-term potentiation, which is a process by, which memories are formed. Animal studies suggest that low levels of thyroid hormones are associated with impairment of long-term potentiation, and thus of memory.

Lab Findings

Tests of individuals with overt thyroid dysfunction show an increase in TSH, low levels of the hormone T4, and/or low levels of the hormone T3. (See Chapter 2 for more about hypothyroidism.)

Effects

In overt hypothyroidism, there is a widespread mild to moderate decrease in cognitive ability. Hypothyroidism can decrease several brain functions, including general intelligence, general memory, the ability to pay attention and concentrate, perceptual function, language ability, psychomotor function (the relationship between brain function and physical movement), executive function (the mental skills that enable the brain to organize and act on information), and verbal memory (the memory of words and other aspects of language).

Test Results

Imaging studies performed on individuals with overt hypothyroidism have provided a good deal of physical evidence that brain function is altered in patients with this condition. Signs of overt hypothyroidism have been shown to include decreased blood flow; decreased function globally (throughout the brain), including areas that are necessary for attention and focus; decreased perception of the spatial relationships between objects in the individual's field of vision; decreased working memory—the system used to store and manage the information needed to learn, reason, and comprehend; and decreased motor speed—the speed at, which body movement takes place.

Treatment

Fortunately, trials have shown that the replacement of T4 is helpful in most patients since it enhances learning ability and recall. For instance, in functional MRI (imaging) studies, hypothyroid individuals with decreased working memory experienced an improvement in memory after being treated with levothyroxine—a synthetic form of the T4 hormone—for 6 months. More studies need to be conducted, as additional patients might have improved if they had been treated with both T4 and T3.

If you are experiencing memory problems or other problems with cognitive function, it is worthwhile to consider the possibility that overt hypothyroidism is the root cause. To learn more about hypothyroidism, turn to Chapter 2, which will fill you in on the disorder's symptoms, methods of diagnosis, and possible forms of treatment, including not just thyroid replacement therapy but also detoxification, supplements, exercise, and diet.

SUBCLINICAL HYPOTHYROIDISM

Subclinical hypothyroidism is a mild form of hypothyroidism (low thyroid function) in, which there are no obvious symptoms of thyroid trouble.

Lab Findings

Laboratory tests reveal only one abnormal hormone level: an increase in TSH or a TSH that is the upper limit of normal. Levels of T3 and T4 are usually within normal ranges. There is strong evidence that subclinical hypothyroidism is associated with a progression to an overt form of this disorder.

Effects

Smaller studies designed to evaluate patients for subtle cognitive impairment have shown that individuals with subclinical hypothyroidism may display mild cognitive changes. The most commonly affected areas were memory and executive function. In one study, patients with subclinical hypothyroidism were shown to have impaired working memory, which means that they had trouble storing and using the information needed to learn, reason, and comprehend. In another study, the authors found that thyroid dysfunction, especially subclinical hypothyroidism, was associated with cognitive impairment. Dementia also increased more with a greater increase in TSH.

Test Results and Treatments

Functional MRI (imaging) studies have shown abnormal function in the frontal brain areas that are responsible for decision-making and planning. Some of the patients were treated with levothyroxine, a synthetic form of T4. This therapy resulted in normal working memory and normal function visible on the MRI.

Furthermore, PET scan imaging revealed that individuals with subclinical hypothyroidism have lower-than-average glucose metabolism in the areas of the brain responsible for cognition. Since glucose is the brain's primary form of fuel, this indicates that subclinical hypothyroidism may compromise brain function, which is dependent on glucose. After 3 months of thyroid replacement therapy with T4, normal metabolic function was restored, enabling the brain to receive the energy it needs.

Although hormone therapy has been shown to help relieve cognitive problems associated with subclinical hypothyroidism, the treatment of this health condition is controversial, particularly when patients do not have recognized symptoms of thyroid disease, such as fatigue, increased sensitivity to cold, and elevated cholesterol levels. (See the inset on page 173 for more about the treatment of subclinical thyroid problems.)

Nevertheless, if you are experiencing cognitive problems, you should consider the possibility that they may be related to a subclinical form of low thyroid function. To learn more, turn to Chapter 2, which will fill you in on methods of diagnosis and possible forms of treatment, including not just thyroid replacement therapy but also detoxification, nutrients, and a healthy eating program.

Subclinical Thyroid Conditions— To Treat or Not to Treat

While most physicians agree that thyroid levels, which are clearly in "abnormal" ranges require treatment, the idea of treating subclinical hypothyroidism (see page 171) or subclinical hyperthyroidism (see page 175) is more controversial. Subclinical thyroid dysfunction is defined as a condition in, which there is an abnormal TSH level—it is too high in hypothyroidism, and too low in hyperthyroidism—but the levels of the T3 and T4 thyroid hormones are within normal ranges. Doctors are especially reluctant to treat these disorders when the patient is not experiencing symptoms that are generally associated with thyroid dysfunction. But some physicians who work with patients who have psychiatric and neurological problems have demonstrated that the treatment of subclinical thyroid conditions can make an important difference, especially in the case of hypothyroidism.

In a study published in 2006, researchers in China provided patients who had subclinical hypothyroidism with levothyroxine therapy. Brain scans used before and after treatment showed significant improvements in both memory and executive function. Confirming these findings are anecdotal reports of psychiatrists who have had good results in treating people whose symptoms were often debilitating—even though their hypothyroidism was considered relatively minor. In fact, results of thyroid hormone therapy have been so encouraging that a few years after the study in China, researchers at Boston University began a trial to explore the connection between subclinical hypothyroidism and certain mood and cognitive disorders.

Begin et al. explained that subclinical hypothyroidism could be a predisposing factor for cognitive impairment. Their review showed that people who had subclinical hypothyroidism for 16 years or more manifested impaired cognitive activity compared to healthy subjects. Young adult patients with subclinical hypothyroidism experienced mild dysfunction in memory, learning, and selective attention.

OVERT HYPERHYROIDISM

Overt hyperthyroidism is hyperthyroidism (higher-than-normal thyroid function) that can be measured by laboratory tests and manifests itself in obvious thyroid symptoms. It occurs when the thyroid gland is overactive and produces too much thyroid hormone, which speeds up the body's metabolism.

Lab Findings

Tests of individuals with overt hyperthyroidism usually show a decrease in TSH and an increase in both T3 and T4 levels, although occasionally, the level of only one of these hormones is higher than normal. (See Chapter 4 for more about hyperthyroidism.)

Effects

Although memory and other cognitive problems seem to be more prevalent among people with hypothyroidism, a number of studies have shown an association between hyperthyroidism and cognitive disorders. People with Graves' disease, the most common cause of hyperthyroidism, are the most likely among hyperthyroid patients to report memory and concentration problems, as well as mood changes. Studies have shown that these symptoms can appear as much as two years earlier than other signs of the disorder. In fact, cognitive problems such as decreased memory and mood changes such as anxiety are often what lead patients to treatment in the first place.

Test Results

The subjective experiences of Graves' patients have been supported by functional imaging studies (PET scans), which have shown cerebral dysfunction, including abnormal glucose metabolism in the right hemispheric limbic system, which is a major region for long-term memory. (To learn more about Graves' disease, see Chapter 5.)

Treatment

In most studies, treatments designed to restore optimal thyroid function have resulted in improved cognition and emotional well-being in people with overt hyperthyroidism. In some studies, however, some residual attention deficits have remained even after the thyroid hormones were being produced in normal amounts.

If you are experiencing memory problems, attention problems, or mood changes, recognize that they may be caused by hyperthyroidism. To learn more about this condition, turn to Chapter 4, which will fill you in on the disorder's symptoms, methods of diagnosis, and possible forms of treatment, including medication, surgery, radioactive therapy, nutritional supplements, and diet. Be aware, though, that if you have Graves' disease and your symptoms include emotional changes, such as nervousness, restlessness, and anxiety, your physician may conclude that you have a psychiatric problem such as generalized anxiety disorder. Too often, patients with Graves' disease are misdiagnosed because of these symptoms, causing delays in a true diagnosis and appropriate treatment. Make sure that your doctor performs the laboratory tests necessary to fully assess the reason for your condition.

SUBCLINICAL HYPERTHYROIDISM

Subclinical hyperthyroidism is a mild form of hyperthyroidism (higher than-normal thyroid function) in, which there are no obvious symptoms. Early Graves' disease, discussed above, accounts for the majority of subclinical hyperthyroidism cases. It has been found that few people with subclinical hyperthyroidism progress to an overt form of the disease.

Lab Findings

Laboratory tests reveal only one abnormal level: a decrease in TSH. Levels of T3 and T4 are within normal ranges.

Effects

The possible relationship between subclinical hyperthyroidism and cognitive problems is a controversial subject. Some studies show a connection, and some do not. Major cognitive problems are not usually seen, but mild problems with memory and concentration may be present. There is some evidence, too, that subclinical hyperthyroidism may be associated with an increased risk of developing dementia, but again, the findings have been conflicting. Subclinical hyperthyroidism appears to be more common in the elderly than it is in younger people.

Treatment

As explained earlier in the chapter, the treatment of subclinical thyroid problems is a subject of debate among doctors, especially when the individual doesn't have recognized symptoms of the disorder. (See the inset on page 173.) Nevertheless, if you are experiencing cognitive problems, a possible thyroid dysfunction should be investigated. Be aware, too, that subclinical hyperthyroidism can indicate the overuse of thyroid hormones. In fact, this disorder is present in about 20 to 40 percent of subjects prescribed thyroid hormones and may indicate overtreatment. So, if you are on thyroid replacement therapy for *hypo*thyroidism and are experiencing cognitive or mood problems, it is a good idea to contact your doctor about the possible need to adjust your medication dose.

HASHIMOTO'S ENCEPHALOPATHY

Hashimoto's encephalopathy (HE) is a disease that involves impaired brain function (encephalopathy). The condition is named for its possible association with Hashimoto's thyroiditis, a common autoimmune thyroid disease, but the exact cause is not totally understood. Hashimoto's encephalopathy is considered rare, affecting just two people out of every 100,000. However, it has been suggested in the medical literature that many more cases are undiagnosed or misdiagnosed since the condition is not easily recognized. The average age of onset of symptoms of Hashimoto's encephalopathy is between 40 to 55 years old. Women are diagnosed with it about four times more often than men. This disorder can also affect children but is thought to be rare.

Lab Findings

No specific diagnostic tests are available to detect Hashimoto's encephalopathy. The presence of some autoantibodies has been reported. In about 75 percent of reported cases, samples of the cerebrospinal fluid revealed an elevated level of proteins, but in 25 percent of the cases, this indicator is not present.

Effects

The symptoms of Hashimoto's encephalopathy are primarily neurological. Among them are memory and concentration problems as well as disorientation, seizures, tremor, myoclonus (rapid contraction and relaxation of muscles), and ataxia (lack of muscle control during voluntary movements, such as walking or picking up objects).

Test Results

Electroencephalography (EEG)—a record of electrical activity of the brain—is usually abnormal. This disease is difficult to detect, and diagnosis is usually performed through a process of exclusion.

Treatment

The treatment for Hashimoto's encephalopathy is steroid therapy, and rapid improvement can usually be observed within one to three days. Although this disorder is thyroid-related, it does not respond to thyroid therapy.

CONCLUSION

Optimal thyroid function is required for perfect focus and memory. As you have seen in this chapter, if thyroid hormone function is too high or too low, the condition may cause a decrease in focus and cognitive decline. It's important to recognize, too, that thyroid function imbalances, which are allowed to continue without treatment can result in more serious health disorders over time. In a long-term trial that was part of the Framingham Study, it was found that women having either high or low levels of TSH had an increased risk of developing Alzheimer's disease, a degenerative disease for, which there is no cure. Consequently, whenever cognitive problems are experienced, thyroid function should be checked and, if a problem is found, appropriate treatment should be initiated. In most cases this results in improved memory, focus, and overall brain function.

8

Thyroid Dysfunction and Your Mood

As you learned in Chapter 7, thyroid problems can affect the brain, which, in turn, can have an adverse effect on mental functions, such as the ability to create and preserve memory. Chapter 7 also touched on the fact that by acting on brain function, thyroid dysfunction can have an impact on mood changes, such as anxiety and depression. This chapter shines a spotlight on the link between the thyroid disorders and mental disorders. Neuropsychiatric disorders account for approximately 14 percent of the global burden of disease.

The relationship between thyroid function and mood has been recognized for many years. However, it is only recently that methodology such as functional neuroimaging has been available to facilitate investigation of thyroid hormone metabolism. Thyroid hormones are widely distributed in the brain and have a multitude of effects on the central nervous system. Notably many of the limbic system structures where thyroid hormone receptors are prevalent have been implicated in the pathogenesis of mood disorders. Thyroid hormone also plays an important role in the release of neurotransmitters, therefore thyroid hormone dysfunction can cause neurotransmitter imbalances.

This chapter first explores neurotransmitters, the chemical messengers that not only send messages within the brain, but also have a profound effect on our emotional well-being. Abnormalities in neurotransmitter release and activity have been linked to various diseases, particularly neuropsychiatric and neurodegenerative disorders. The influence of the thyroid system on neurotransmitters (particularly serotonin and norepinephrine), which putatively play a major role in the regulation of mood and behavior, may contribute to the mechanisms of mood modulation.

This section of the book then takes a closer look at both depression and anxiety. Generally, an overactive thyroid (hyperthyroidism) can lead to anxiety, as well as nervousness, restlessness, and irritability. An underactive thyroid (hypothyroidism) is more likely to lead to depression. The more severe the thyroid disorder, the more severe the mood changes are likely to be.

NEUROTRANSMITTERS

The brain is composed of over 100 billion nerve cells called neurons. It is through the neurons that the brain passes on information (or signals) that allow you to recognize and react physically and emotionally to both your internal thoughts and external stimuli, such as heat and cold. Every time you respond to an event or a feeling, every time you feel happy or sad, it is because of this system of message transmission.

Since neurons do not touch each other physically, but are separated by gaps called synapses, the messages (which are electrochemical signals) cannot move directly from one neuron to another. Instead, chemical neurotransmitters bridge the gaps, passing on the information from cell to cell. This happens very quickly, with millions of neurons being affected in an instant.

The brain produces two basic types of neurotransmitters.

- **Excitatory neurotransmitters.** These neurotransmitters promote the transmission of information from one neuron to another and have a stimulating effect on the body. They include aspartic acid, epinephrine (also known as adrenaline), glutamate, histamine, norepinephrine, and PEA (phenylethylamine).

- **Inhibitory neurotransmitters.** These neurotransmitters decrease the ability to transmit messages and have a calming effect on the body. These chemicals include agmatine, GABA (gamma-aminobutyric acid), glycine, serotonin, and taurine.

- **Dopamine.** This is a unique neurotransmitter in that it is both inhibitory and excitatory.

Each of the substances just named regulates specific functions in the body. The list beginning on page 181 gives you a clearer idea of the amazingly varied tasks that these vital chemicals perform, as well as symptoms of neurotransmitter deficiency, and the foods that can increase production of each of these important chemicals.

As the following list shows, in addition to performing a myriad of other functions, several neurotransmitters regulate mood. Serotonin is known as the "happy" neurotransmitter. When serotonin levels decrease in the body, feelings of depression, anxiety, or agitation may occur. Dopamine is another neurotransmitter that provides feelings of pleasure and enjoyment. GABA, histamine, and PEA also help regulate mood. It's important to understand, though, that *all* of the neurotransmitters are required for emotional well-being, as they interact with each other and with other chemicals in the body to maintain both physical and mental health. When the body produces the correct amount of these chemicals and they are in balance, your mood is positive, and you feel upbeat and calm. When neurotransmitter levels are too high or too low, you can become depressed or anxious.

NEUROTRANSMITTER FUNCTION AND DEFICIENCY

AGMATINE

Functions

- Aids wound healing
- Enhances immune function
- Enhances metabolism of fats
- Helps build proteins
- Helps produce glucagon and insulin
- Increases circulation
- Increases production of growth hormone
- Increases sperm count
- Inhibits accumulation of plaque in the arteries
- Needed for digestive health
- Reduces pain from poor circulation

Symptoms of Deficiency

- Agmatine deficiency is rare because the amino acid used in its manufacture is found in many foods and also made in the body.

Foods That Can Increase Agmatine Levels in the Body: Avocados; Beans; Brewer's yeast; Corn; Dark chocolate; Eggs; Green vegetables such as asparagus, broccoli, peas, and spinach; Meat; Dairy products; Nuts; Oatmeal; Onions; Potatoes; Raisins; Seafood; Seeds; Soy; and Whole grains.

ASPARTIC ACID

Functions

- Aids energy production from carbohydrate metabolism
- Assists production of DNA and RNA
- Enhances immune system function
- Helps protect the liver from drug toxicity
- Increases energy and endurance

Symptoms of Deficiency

- Depression
- Fatigue
- Reduced stamina

Foods That Can Increase Aspartic Acid Levels in the Body: Meat, Poultry, and Seafood.

DOPAMINE

Functions

- Controls the body's movements
- Maintains good concentration, memory, and problem-solving
- Provides feeling of enjoyment and pleasure, reinforcing certain behaviors
- Regulates flow of information to other parts of the brain
- Stabilizes brain activity

Symptoms of Deficiency

- Depression
- Excessive sleeping
- Inability to experience pleasure
- Tendency to crave and eat junk food, especially sweets
- Tendency to form addictions

Foods That Can Increase Dopamine Levels in the Body: Almonds, Avocados, Bananas, Beans, Dairy products, Poultry (especially turkey), Pumpkin seeds, Seafood (especially salmon), and Sesame seeds.

EPINEPHRINE (ADRENALINE)

Functions

- Constricts arteries
- Opens airways in lungs
- Quickens heartbeat
- Raises blood pressure
- Regulates blood pressure
- Regulates mental focus
- Strengthens force of heart's contractions
- Triggers release of glucose from energy stores

Symptoms of Deficiency

- Addison's disease
- Allergies
- Constipation
- Decreased tolerance to cold
- Depression or apathy
- Fatigue
- Low blood pressure
- Low blood sugar
- Muscle weakness
- Need for excessive sleep
- Poor circulation

Foods That Can Increase Epinephrine Levels in the Body: Beans, Dairy products, Eggs, Meat, Poultry, Tofu, and Seafood.

GABA

Functions

- Acts as muscle relaxant
- Calms the brain
- Lowers blood pressure
- Prevents anxiety
- Promotes secretion of growth hormone
- Relieves stress

Symptoms of Deficiency

- Anxiety
- Insomnia
- Rapid heartbeat
- Seizures
- Sensation that brain is racing out of control

Foods That Can Increase GABA Levels in the Body: Beans, Brewer's yeast, Dairy products, Eggs, Fish, Legumes, Meat, Nuts, Seafood, Seeds, Soy, and Whole grains.

GLUTAMATE

Functions

- Balances blood sugar
- Decreases food cravings
- Enhances pain control
- Enhances sensory perception
- Fuels the immune system
- Improves mental alertness
- Increases energy
- Maintains digestive health
- Maintains muscle health

- Neutralizes toxins
- Plays a part in sensory perception
- Promotes healing
- Promotes healthy acid-alkaline balance
- Promotes weight loss
- Supports memory
- Supports motor skills

Symptoms of Deficiency

- Glutamate deficiency is rare because this substance is found in many foods and manufactured in the body.

Foods That Can Increase Glutamate Levels in the Body: Beans, Brewer's yeast, Brown rice, Dairy products, Eggs, Fish, Meat, Nuts, Seafood, Seeds, Soy, and Whole grains.

GLYCINE

Functions

- Aids absorption of calcium
- Aids in production of ATP, which stores energy within the cells
- Calms aggression
- Decreases sugar cravings
- Helps build hemoglobin, proteins, DNA, and RNA

- Helps detoxify heavy metals in the body
- Helps maintain the nervous system
- Needed to make bile acids
- Needed to make glutathione, the body's most abundant natural antioxidant
- Promotes healthy prostate gland function

Symptoms of Deficiency

- Glycine deficiency is rare because this substance is found in many foods and manufactured in the body.

Foods That Can Increase Glycine Levels in the Body: Beans, Dairy products, Meat, and Seafood.

HISTAMINE

Functions

- Plays role in development of organs

- Regulates mood

- Signals immune system to react to allergens, causing an inflammatory response

Symptoms of Deficiency

- Depression
- Hallucination
- Paranoia

Foods That Can Increase Histamine Levels in the Body: Citrus fruits, such as oranges and grapefruit; Garlic; Leafy green vegetables, such as spinach; and Onions.

High histamine levels can cause the following symptoms:

- Nasal congestion
- Rosacea
- Irritated eyes
- Insomnia
- Hives
- Itching
- Asthma
- Chronic fatigue
- Diarrhea and other gastrointestinal symptoms
- Brain fog
- Anxiety

High histamine foods and drinks include the following:

- Aged cheese
- Shellfish
- Alcohol and other fermented beverages
- Avocados
- Eggplant
- Spinach
- Processed or smoked meats
- Fermented foods and dairy products such as sauerkraut and yogurt
- Dried fruit

Foods and drinks that trigger a histamine release include:

- Chocolate
- Alcohol
- Bananas
- Tomatoes
- Wheat germ
- Papaya
- Beans
- Citrus fruits
- Nuts such as cashews, peanuts, and walnuts
- Food dyes and other additives

NOREPINEPHRINE

Functions

- Constricts arteries
- Enhances attention and focus
- Increases blood flow to the muscles and brain
- Opens airways in lungs
- Quickens heartbeat
- Raises blood pressure
- Regulates mental focus
- Triggers release of glucose from energy stores

Symptoms of Deficiency

- Depression
- Droopy eyelids
- Fatigue

Foods That Can Increase Norepinephrine Levels in the Body: Beans, Eggs, Meat, Dairy products, Poultry, Seafood, and Tofu.

PHENYLETHYLAMINE (PEA)

Functions

- Elevates mood
- Enhances concentration
- Increases energy
- Promotes mental alertness

Symptoms of Deficiency

- Agitation
- Confusion
- Decreased alertness
- Decreased sexual interest
- Depression
- Fatigue
- Memory problems

Foods That Can Increase Phenylethylamine Levels in the Body: Bananas, Dairy products, Dark chocolate, and Eggs. Do not eat foods that increase PEA if you have PKU.

SEROTONIN

Functions

- Calms anxiety
- Controls appetite and carbohydrate cravings
- Regulates body temperature
- Regulates sexual behavior
- Regulates sleep cycles
- Relieves depression

Symptoms of Deficiency

- Anxiety
- Cravings for sugar
- Depression
- Fatigue
- Insomnia
- Loss of concentration
- Poor impulse control

Foods That Can Increase Serotonin Levels in the Body: Beef, Chickpeas, Dairy products, Dates, Eggs, Peanuts, Poultry, Seafood, and Sunflower seeds.

TAURINE

Functions

- Aids glucose metabolism
- Aids wound healing
- Boosts immune function
- Enhances use of calcium
- Important for brain and nervous system function
- Important for visual pathways
- Improves insulin sensitivity
- Improves liver function
- Improves lung function
- Lowers blood pressure
- Lowers cholesterol
- Prevents blood clots
- Promotes kidney function
- Protects against cell membrane damage
- Stabilizes heart rhythms
- Strengthens the heart muscle

Symptoms of Deficiency

- Anxiety
- Depression
- High blood pressure
- Hyperactivity
- Hypothyroidism (low thyroid function)

- Impaired vision
- Infertility

- Kidney dysfunction
- Seizures

Foods That Can Increase Taurine Levels in the Body: Brewer's yeast, Dairy products, Eggs, Fish, Meat, and Seafood. Avoid foods that contain MSG, since MSG degrades taurine.

NEUROTRANSMITTERS AND THE THYROID

What is the relationship between neurotransmitters and the thyroid? Several studies have shown that low levels of thyroid hormones lead to low levels of neurotransmitters, including those neurotransmitters that have been shown to influence mood. For instance, low thyroid hormones can cause a decreased production of the neurotransmitter dopamine, leading to depression and the loss of motivation and willpower. Insufficient production of thyroid hormones can also decrease the levels of GABA and serotonin—two other neurotransmitters vital to the regulation of mood.

Further studies are needed to explain the complex interaction between the thyroid, the neurotransmitter system, and your emotions. For the time being, if you think you are experiencing the symptoms of neurotransmitter dysfunction, the only way to know for sure is to see a healthcare provider that specializes in Anti-Aging/Personalized Medicine. (See Resources on page 329.) This specialist can arrange for urine tests that can detect neurotransmitters and their metabolites. In addition, try to improve your diet to include some of the healthy neurotransmitter-stimulating foods listed on pages 181 to 188. Finally, consider the possibility that your thyroid hormone production may be low or high and affecting the levels of your mood-balancing neurotransmitters. Below, you'll learn more about the relationship between thyroid dysfunction, depression, and anxiety.

DEPRESSION

Depression is the most common mental health condition, reportedly affecting one in ten Americans at some point in their lives. More than 21 million people in the United States are estimated to have had at least one major depressive episode. Consequently, this illness has been called the "common cold" of mental health disorders. Moreover, it is rapidly becoming a significant health concern worldwide. Mood disorders, including major depressive disorder (MDD) and bipolar disorder (BD), have a global lifetime prevalence of up to 20 percent. Indeed, both hypo- and hyperthyroidism have been associated with MDD and/or BD in observational studies. In addition, a recent study revealed that subclinical hypothyroidism has a negative impact on depression. Early and routine screening of depression is essential to prevent morbidity and mortality. This screening demands an adequate evaluation of thyroid function where all of your thyroid studies are measured.

What Is Depression?

Depression is a medical disorder that involves both the mind and the body. Far more than a case of the blues, it is a feeling of unhappiness, melancholy, or despair that lasts for a prolonged period of time—weeks, months, or even years. It often recurs over time, requiring long-term treatment, just like diabetes or heart disease.

Although depression is sometimes thought of as being extreme sadness, there is a big difference between sadness and clinical depression, which is also called major depression and major depressive disorder. Everyone experiences sadness at some time in their lives, usually as the result of unpleasant circumstances, such as the loss of a job or the death of a loved one. In time, the sadness lifts as the individual deals with life's problems. But in the case of clinical depression, the feelings last much longer and the individual often does not know their cause. Furthermore, while people who are sad usually manage to cope with life and perform everyday activities, those who are clinically depressed may feel overwhelmed and unable to deal with common tasks. Moreover, depression usually includes some symptoms—such as backache—that are not associated with a temporary case of the blues.

What are the Symptoms of Depression?

The symptoms of depression can vary from person to person, and also according to age. Below, you will find the signs and symptoms that are characteristic of adult depression. Following this, you will find symptoms of depression that are specific to certain age groups. Be aware that older adults may also have the common signs of adult depression, but that some of these problems—fatigue, loss of appetite, and reduced interest in sex, for example—typically go unrecognized because they are seen as being part of aging or another illness. It is important to recognize *all* behaviors and feelings to determine if you or someone you know may be suffering from depression.

Common Symptoms of Adult Depression

- Agitation or restlessness, resulting in hand-wringing or pacing

- Crying spells without cause

- Decreased appetite and weight loss

- Increased appetite and weight gain

- Excessive sleeping

- Fatigue

- Feelings of sadness

- Feelings of worthlessness or guilt

- Frequent thoughts of death or suicide

- Frustration and irritability, even over small events

- Indecisiveness

- Insomnia

- Intense cravings for certain foods

- Loss of concentration

- Loss of interest in activities that are normally pleasurable

- Reduced sex drive

- Slowness in thinking, speaking, or moving

- Unexplained physical problems such as backache

Symptoms Characteristic of Adolescent and Teen Depression

- Anxiety and anger

- Avoidance of social situations

- Behavior and mental health problems such as attention deficit hyperactivity disorder (ADHD)

Symptoms Characteristic of Older Adult Depression

- Desire to stay home

- Feelings of boredom and dissatisfaction with life

- Thoughts of suicide

What Is the Treatment for Depression?

A combination of treatments may be used to relieve depression. Treatment may include various types of antidepressants and/or some form of psychotherapy, such as cognitive therapy, interpersonal therapy, behavioral therapy, or problem-solving therapy. Although a depressive disorder can be debilitating, hindering the individual's ability to work, sleep, and eat, only about half of Americans who have major depression receive help. Many people resist treatment because they believe that the condition isn't serious, that they can manage it themselves, or that the disorder is a sign of personal weakness. This is unfortunate, as about 70 percent of those who seek medical help experience significant improvement and depression is just like any other illness such as hypertension or diabetes. It has nothing to do with personal weakness.

Of course, to a large degree, successful treatment depends on understanding the cause of the depression. If the root cause is thyroid dysfunction, that problem must be resolved in order to restore emotional well-being.

Depression and Thyroid Dysfunction

Depression has long been known to be a common symptom of hypothyroidism, or low thyroid function. See Chapter 2 for more about hypothyroidism. In fact, even subclinical (undetected) hypothyroidism—a relatively mild form of the disease, in, which no obvious signs of thyroid problems are seen—has been found present in up to 40 percent of patients with depression. It is believed that hypothyroidism can lead to depression in several ways.

- As you learned earlier in the chapter, hypothyroidism can cause this condition by decreasing the production of neurotransmitters. Neurotransmitters such as serotonin, dopamine, and GABA are needed in optimal amounts to maintain emotional health. When thyroid function is abnormally low, it causes levels of these chemicals to drop, and depression can result.

- Hypothyroidism can also influence mood by affecting the mitochondria, which are the cell structures that create energy. Thyroid hormones are essential for both the formation and the function of the mitochondria, so when thyroid function is insufficient, fatigue, depression, and foggy thinking can result.

- Thyroid dysfunction can also cause depression by affecting the balance of a myriad of hormones, including estrogen, progesterone, testosterone, DHEA, pregnenolone, and cortisol. Hormone imbalance prevents the body from managing stress and experiencing positive moods.

- Depression is known to be associated with changes in the hypothalamic-pituitary-thyroid (HPT) axis. The hypothalamus-pituitary-thyroid (HPT) axis determines the set point of thyroid hormone production. Hypothalamic thyrotropin-releasing hormone (TRH) stimulates the synthesis and secretion of pituitary thyrotropin (thyroid-stimulating hormone, TSH), which acts on the thyroid to stimulate all steps of thyroid hormone biosynthesis and secretion. The thyroid hormones thyroxine (T4) and triiodothyronine (T3) control the secretion of TRH and TSH by a negative feedback mechanism, which maintains physiological levels of the main hormones of the HPT axis. Furthermore, reduction of circulating thyroid hormone levels due to primary thyroid failure results in increased thyroid releasing hormone and TSH production, whereas the opposite occurs when circulating thyroid hormones are in excess.

- Depression has been linked to various endogenous circadian rhythms abnormalities, such as diurnal mood variation (depression symptoms that are worse in the morning and improve as the day progresses), abnormalities in core body temperature, cortisol (stress hormone) secretion, and sleep-wake cycle. In addition to these circadian dysfunctions, depression has been linked to an abnormal diurnal (daytime) TSH rhythm as well. An absent TSH nocturnal (nighttime) surge has been noted in depression and a lower basal TSH has been reported in major depression as opposed to non-major depression. Furthermore, a blunted TSH response to TRH was reported in about 25 to 3percent of depressed subjects compared to healthy ones. One major hypothesis to explain the above finding is that chronic TRH hypersecretion is associated with depression, which leads to downregulation of pituitary TRH receptors.

- One mechanism explaining the increase in T4 seen in depression is the activation of hypothalamic TRH producing neurons and subsequent increase in thyroid function secondary to the rise in cortisol associated with depression. In addition, it has been shown that elevated serum T4 levels fall after successful treatment of depression. A direct effect of antidepressants on the TRH neuron has been demonstrated resulting in an inhibition of TRH secretion. This suggests that the decrease in T4 levels with initiation of antidepressants could be secondary to a direct effect on TRH neurons and thus to a reduced stimulation of the thyroid axis.

According to the American Association of Clinical Endocrinologists, whenever a patient is diagnosed with a depressive disorder, subclinical or clinical hypothyroidism should be considered. In fact, the link between these two disorders is so well known that thyroid medications—such as liothyronine (synthetic T3 hormone) and levothyroxine (synthetic T4 hormone)—are sometimes added to antidepressant treatment, even when thyroid function has been found normal in laboratory tests. The goal here is to optimize thyroid function.

The Sequenced Treatment Alternatives to Relieve Depression (STAR*D) study showed that the combination of T3 thyroid hormone and antidepressants resulted in additional improvements in about 25 percent of subjects whose major depression had not been relieved by antidepressant therapy alone. This phenomenon is believed to be due to one of two theories. One theory is that thyroid drugs and antidepressants work synergistically to boost each other's effects. Another possibility is that thyroid hormone replacement stimulates chemical activity in the brain, enhancing both mood and concentration. Whatever the mechanism involved, it is clear that when depression is a problem, and especially when standard treatments provide little if any improvement, the possibility of thyroid dysfunction should be explored. In addition, thyroid hormone supplementation may have a role in the treatment of mood disorders, particularly rapid-cycling bipolar disorder.

Another study revealed that functional brain imaging studies using positron emission tomography (PET) demonstrated that thyroid hormone treatment with levothyroxine affects regional brain metabolism in individuals with hypothyroidism and bipolar disorder. These studies confirm that thyroid hormones are active in modulating metabolic function in the mature adult brain and provide intriguing clues that may guide research in the future.

Subclinical Hypothyroidism

Subclinical hypothyroidism is defined as an elevated thyroid stimulating hormone (TSH) with normal free T4 and free T3 levels. It affects 3 percent to 8.5 percent of the general population with a female preponderance, and a higher rate up to 20 percent among elderly people. Traditionally, depression is reported among people aged 35 to 45 years. Of note, it has become increasingly common in the elderly as normal aging itself is associated with biochemical changes in the HPT (hypothalamic-pituitary-thyroid) axis. The secretion of thyroid hormones is commonly reduced with increasing age, with a lower free T3 level, but a relatively unchanged free T4 concentration. Compared with the younger population, higher TSH level is seen in the elderly due to reduced free T4 breakdown and its peripheral conversion to free T3, with subsequent positive feedback to the HPT axis.

As you have seen, individuals with overt hypothyroidism experience a wide variety of clinical signs and symptoms, including cold intolerance, weight gain, cognitive dysfunction, and mood disturbances. It is important to note that only up to 30 percent of individuals with subclinical hypothyroidism share similar clinical features with the elderly group who experience even fewer and less recognizable complaints. This may result in a delayed diagnosis of subclinical hypothyroidism. Given the aging population in the world and an increased risk of depression in the elderly with subclinical hypothyroidism, there is an urgent need for TSH and depression screening in this vulnerable population, in order to improve well-being and to help a person achieve optimal health.

Although one study showed no significant difference in the serum TSH level between individuals with depression and healthy controls, this could possibly be a phenomenon known as the "brain hypothyroidism," which represents a low intracerebral (occurring in the cerebrum of the brain) free T3 concentration with normal peripheral thyroid hormones and TSH levels. Physiologically, as discussed in chapter 1, type II deiodinase converts free T4 to free T3 in the brain glial cells. However, it has been postulated that depression can cause an inhibitory effect on type II deiodinase, which leads to the conversion of free T4 to reverse T3 (rT3) via type III deiodinase. Furthermore, transthyretin, a serum transport protein for free T4 in cerebrospinal fluid, is reduced in individuals with refractory depression. Ultimately, these affects result in decreased intracerebral free T3 and free T4 levels, along with a high rT3 concentration in cerebrospinal fluid (fluid that surrounds the brain and spinal cord) that can also inactivate free T3 activity. Therefore, some patients may improve with adding nutrients to lower reverse T3. (See page 20.)

In addition, some people have not been shown to have their depression improved with levothyroxine (T4). Given the reduced activity of intracerebral type II deiodinase in depression, levothyroxine therapy might be converted to rT3 that could exacerbate the existing intracerebral free T3 deficiency. This has been called "low T3 syndrome." In a small trial of nine individuals with refractory depression, on top of antidepressant and levothyroxine (T4) therapy, additional administration of liothyronine (T3) was associated with marked improvement in the symptoms of depression in seven of them.

Further studies, which examine the variations between intracerebral and peripheral thyroid hormones and TSH levels in different populations are needed to have a better understanding of this very important relationship.

Autoimmune Thyroid Disorders

There are trials revealing that anti-thyroid antibodies are involved in the development of depression. A prevalence of up to 20 percent of elevated titers of antithyroid antibodies has been documented in depressed patients in several reports compared to 5 percent to 10 percent prevalence in the general population. Consequently, the prevalence of depression is significantly higher in patients with Hashimoto's thyroiditis than in the general population. Moreover, free T3, free T4, and TSH are dysregulated, and free T4 has the potential to serve as an independent biomarker for predicting anxiety as well as depression in autoimmune disorder patients.

Furthermore, nowadays, the gravity of psychiatric disorders in patients with all autoimmune disorders has been increasingly explored, and studies report that individuals with many autoimmune disorders present with a higher risk of developing anxiety and depression. Moreover, anxiety and depression are factors that impair not only the quality of life but also recovery from whichever autoimmune disorder that you may have.

Additionally, the association of postpartum depression with postpartum thyroiditis or with positive thyroid antibodies is still not well defined. Early studies noted a minor association between thyroid dysfunction and postnatal depression. More recently, a higher frequency of mild to moderate depression was observed in postpartum female subjects with positive antithyroid antibodies regardless of thyroid function.

Thyroid Hormone Replacement Therapy

Thyroid hormone replacement has been used as an adjunct to antidepressant therapy since the late 1960s to accelerate clinical response to antidepressants and to increase the likelihood of a response from non-responders to antidepressants, which is called augmentation therapy. Moreover, an acceleration of antidepressant effect by T3 has been initially shown more than 30 years ago in several reports. A meta-analysis of these early double-blind placebo-controlled trials concluded that T3 was effective in accelerating the clinical response to tricyclic antidepressants in individuals with depression that did not response to two antidepressants. The effects of T3 acceleration appeared to be more remarkable as the percentage of women in a trial increased, therefore suggesting that women might benefit more than men from T3 supplementation. In addition, several reports examined the role of T3 as an augmentation strategy to antidepressants in refractory depression. In a study, patients with C785T polymorphism (associated with higher rT3 levels and a lower T3/rT3 ratio) in D1 gene had a better response to T3. Therefore, depressed patients with genetically determined lower T4 to T3 conversion could therefore derive more benefit from thyroid hormone augmentation therapy.

Fewer studies assessed the efficacy of T4 in the treatment of affective disorders. Joffe and Singer found a significantly higher response to tricyclic antidepressants with T3 compared to T4. Clearly, further research is needed to ascertain whether thyroid hormone supplementation may effectively accelerate and potentiate the therapeutic response to antidepressant drugs. In addition, the role of genetic variations in deiodinase enzymes in the response to antidepressant therapy merits further investigation.

Hyperthyroidism

The common view is that clinical hypothyroidism is associated with depressive symptoms, whereas the psychiatric manifestations of hyperthyroidism are agitation, emotional lability, hyperexcitability, anxiety, and occasionally accompanied by angry outbursts, and euphoria. A recent case reported overturns this conventional medical knowledge. A 73-year-old Italian woman experienced a severe major depressive episode with psychotic and melancholic features during laboratory thyrotoxicosis. No classical clinical signs and symptoms of thyrotoxicosis were present. Psychiatric symptoms improved together with treatment of her hyperthyroidism. Recent neuroimaging has provided possible neurobiological explanations, showing how the excess thyroid hormones could affect brain structures involved in the regulation of mood, leading to depression. A direct link between hyperthyroidism and depression seems to be likely according to this case history. Consequently, hyperthyroidism may be associated with depression as well as anxiety.

ANXIETY

Like depression, anxiety is a common mental health condition. In fact, anxiety disorders form the most common group of mental disorders and generally start before or in early adulthood. Main features include excessive fear and anxiety or avoidance of perceived threats that are persistent and impairing. Anxiety disorders involve dysfunction in brain circuits that respond to danger. Risks for anxiety disorders are influenced by genetic factors, environmental factors, and their epigenetic (the study of changes in organisms caused by modification of gene expression rather than alteration of the genetic code itself) relations. Anxiety disorders are often comorbid with one another and with other mental disorders, especially depression. In any given year, some form of anxiety affects about 18 percent of the U.S. population. It is estimated that each year, 40 million Americans experience anxiety symptoms severe enough to disrupt their daily activities, including job performance, schoolwork, and relationships.

What Is Anxiety?

Anxiety is a feeling of worry, nervousness, or unease. Although these are normal human emotions that often occur in times of difficulty, an anxiety disorder is a serious mental illness that persists for an extended period of time and interferes with the ability to lead a normal life. For some people, anxiety can be crippling.

It's important to understand that there are several different types of anxiety disorders. The four major forms are the following:

- Generalized Anxiety Disorder (GAD). Those who have generalized anxiety disorder often experience excessive worry and fear over situations that for most people are not threatening.

- Panic Disorder. Individuals who have panic disorder experience feelings of terror that strike suddenly and repeatedly, usually without warning. Symptoms—which can include sweating, chest pain, irregular heartbeat, and more—can be so severe that the person may feel that they are having a heart attack.

- Social Anxiety Disorder. People with this form of anxiety, which is also called social phobia, experience overwhelming self-consciousness and worry about everyday social situations. This worry is often based on an extreme fear of being judged harshly by the people around them.

- Specific Phobias. Individuals with specific phobias have an intense fear of a particular object or situation such as spiders, thunderstorms, or flying in an airplane. The level of fear is so great that the person often avoids common situations.

What Are the Symptoms of Anxiety?

The symptoms of anxiety can vary from person to person, and, of course, they also vary according to the type of anxiety disorder involved. The Anxiety and Depression Association of America (ADAA) lists the following as general symptoms of anxiety:

- Chest pain or discomfort
- Chills or heat flashes
- Difficulty breathing, such as shortness of breath or the sensation of smothering
- Fear of dying
- Feelings of dizziness, unsteadiness, or lightheadedness
- Feelings of unreality or of being detached from oneself
- Nausea or abdominal distress
- Palpitations, including a pounding heart or accelerated heart rate
- Sweating
- The sensation of choking
- Trembling or shaking

Dr. Billie Sahley in her book, *The Anxiety Epidemic*, describes the following symptoms of anxiety-fear-panic-phobias.

- Feeling a loss of control
- Think you are going insane
- Feeling light-headed, faint
- Unsteady legs
- Having difficulty breathing—unable to take a deep breath
- Fearing a heart attack
- Pounding, skipping, or racing heart
- Experiencing a constant fear of dying
- Stomach pain, diarrhea, constipation, nausea
- Sweating, excessively even when cold
- Headaches, neck and shoulder pain
- Low-back pain
- Feeling tender headed
- Feeling tired, weak, no energy
- Feeling as though you are outside your body

- Mood and emotional swings
- Insomnia
- Sleeping restlessly with or without nightmares
- Experiencing an inability to relax
- Feeling anxious, tense, and/or restlessness
- Having depressing or negative thought patterns
- Needing to have someone near you constantly
- Having a rush of panic or fear, for no reason
- Fearing crowds, breathing with difficulty
- Eating emotionally, food will not go down
- Muscle twitching, muscle spasms
- Inability to remember

- Staying home
- Dry cotton mouth
- Blurred vision
- Cold hands and feet
- Fearing the dark
- Perspiring more than normal
- Flushing of the face
- Constantly passing gas and/or indigestion
- Never feeling full (bottomless stomach)
- Muscle stiffness
- Mental confusion
- Flushes (hot flashes) or chills
- Choking sensations
- Chest pain
- Numbness and tingling of fingers and lips

What Are the Causes of Anxiety?

There are many possible causes of anxiety and phobias including: genetic predisposition, nutritional deficiencies, post-traumatic stress disorder (PTSD), psychological conflicts, grief, food allergies, prolonged pain from injury, toxic metals, childhood separation, rebound from medications, hypoglycemic, lactate buildup in the bloodstream, excessive use of alcohol, sugar, mitochondrial disorders, hyperthyroidism, abnormal levels of estrogen, progesterone, testosterone, pregnenolone, DHEA, and/or cortisol, and neurotransmitter deficiencies.

What Are the Treatments for Anxiety?

Anxiety disorders are very treatable, and, like depression, a variety of treatments may be used depending on the cause of the disorder. The most common methods of treatment are medications, including traditional anti-anxiety drugs, antidepressants, and beta-blockers; and psychotherapy, such as cognitive behavioral therapy. Only about a third of people with anxiety disorders seek treatment. However, most cases of anxiety disorder—even severe cases—can be treated successfully, with most people feeling substantial relief within a few months. Selective serotonin reuptake inhibitors (SSRIs), serotonin-norepinephrine reuptake inhibitors (SNRIs), benzodiazepines, tricyclic antidepressants, mild tranquilizers, and beta-blockers have been used to treat anxiety disorders.

Alternative approaches, such as biofeedback and calming herbs, are also very useful. If allergies are the cause of your symptoms, then avoiding foods and drinks you are allergic to is beneficial. Having your healthcare provider measure your neurotransmitters and balancing them, if they are abnormal, may be helpful. If your toxic metals load is high, then chelation therapy may resolve some of the anxiety. If the etiology of your anxiety is a mitochondrial problem, then refueling your body with mitochondrial nutrients will help. These are the same nutrients that are beneficial to lower reverse T3 level listed on page 20. In addition, have your healthcare provider order a salivary test to determine if your estrogen, progesterone, testosterone, DHEA, and/or cortisol levels are optimal. Balancing any, or all, of these hormones will definitely help with anxiety in both men and women.

Anxiety and Thyroid Function

As you learned in Chapter 4, hyperthyroidism occurs when the thyroid gland overproduces thyroid hormone. Anxiety is considered one of the most common symptoms of an overactive thyroid. Anxiety disorders have been found to occur in approximately 60 percent of hyperthyroid patients while depressive disorders occurred in 31 percent to 69 percent.

How does hyperthyroidism cause anxiety? Because thyroid hormones activate the entire body, an overproduction of these hormones causes the nervous system to be more active, potentially causing nervous tremors and shaking, sleeplessness, a racing heart, and irritability—all of, which are symptoms of anxiety. This is why it's often difficult to tell the difference between true anxiety and hyperthyroidism.

As explained earlier in the chapter, hyperthyroidism can also cause mood disorders by upsetting the balance of your neurotransmitters, the chemicals that send messages within the brain and also help regulate mood. The function of chemical neurotransmitters is intimately affected by your body's hormones, and when levels of thyroid hormones are too high, neurotransmitter production is disrupted, potentially causing anxiety.

Although we don't know all the ways hyperthyroidism is associated with anxiety, studies have found that an overproduction of thyroid hormones is the most frequent medical condition misdiagnosed as anxiety disorder. This means that in cases of anxiety, the possibility of an overactive thyroid should always be considered.

CONCLUSION

The relation between thyroid function and depression has long been recognized. Because the thyroid gland affects every cell in the body, thyroid function has an influence on every body function. Small wonder, then, that when the thyroid malfunctions, your mood can suffer.

Individuals with thyroid disorders are more prone to develop depressive symptoms and conversely depression may be accompanied by various subtle thyroid abnormalities. Traditionally, the most commonly documented abnormalities are elevated T4 levels, low T3, elevated rT3, a blunted TSH response to TRH, positive antithyroid antibodies, and elevated CSF TRH concentrations. Contact your healthcare provider to see if being prescribed T4 and/or T3 would be beneficial. Furthermore, if reverse T3 is elevated, nutritional therapies may also be helpful. In addition, thyroid hormone replacement appears to accelerate and enhance the clinical response to antidepressant drugs. Recently, hyperthyroidism has also been shown to be related to depression. Consequently, it is imperative that if you are suffering from depression, that your doctor measure all your thyroid hormones to determine if thyroid dysfunction is the cause of your depression.

Moreover, anxiety has also been shown to be related to both hyper and hypothyroidism. If you are experiencing anxiety, it makes sense to request tests designed to detect thyroid problems.

Remember that it is not uncommon for thyroid dysfunction to be misdiagnosed as a disorder with psychological rather than physical roots. Treatments that restore normal function of the thyroid gland, whether used alone or in combination with other therapies, may help to restore your emotional well-being.

9

Thyroid Hormones and Your Heart

There are many reasons why people experience health issues related to their heart—lack of exercise, eating the wrong foods, and a family history of heart troubles to name a few. Moreover, it has been discovered that common signs and symptoms of thyroid disease may be a result of how the thyroid affects the heart and the cardiovascular system. For example, if you have been diagnosed with hyperthyroidism (see Chapters 4 and 5 for details describing hyperthyroidism) and experiencing frequent palpitations or a high heart rate, these heart issues may be directly associated with this condition. In fact, heart related disorders can be associated with an undiagnosed or untreated thyroid dysfunction with hypo or hyperthyroidism. As the evidence will show, thyroid hormone balance is necessary for optimal heart function!

The thyroid is the body regulator, and therefore it is crucial that the thyroid gland functions perfectly and not just normally to help prevent and treat cardiovascular disease. Thyroid disorders can directly affect the normal function of the heart resulting in serious symptoms and cardiac complications. Therefore, thyroid dysfunction as hypothyroidism, or hyperthyroidism, can both have a negative impact upon cardiovascular health and are risk factors for heart disease. It is important to remember that thyroid hormones T4 and T3 are important managers of cardiac function and cardiovascular blood flow.

In addition, it has long been recognized that some of the most characteristic and common signs and symptoms of thyroid disease are those that result from the effects of thyroid hormone on the heart and cardiovascular system. Both hyperthyroidism and hypothyroidism produce changes in cardiac contractility, myocardial oxygen consumption, cardiac output, blood pressure, and systemic vascular resistance (SVR). In almost all cases these cardiovascular changes are reversible when the underlying thyroid disorder is recognized and treated.

This chapter provides you with an overall look at the importance of thyroid hormones and a healthy thyroid gland for peak function of your heart. Presented are the symptoms of a dysfunctional thyroid, how hypothyroidism and hyperthyroidism can affect the heart, and cardiovascular risk factors associated with a thyroid gland that is not functioning optimally. In addition, this chapter will offer a number of important tests and effective treatments.

IMPORTANCE OF T4 AND T3

A healthy heart and cardiovascular system are highly dependent on your having sufficient levels of T3 in your body. This active hormone regulates your metabolism, clearing out excess arterial fatty deposits. T4 is largely considered by many researchers to be an inactive prohormone; that is, it is precursor to another hormone it will turn into. Most of the T4 produced by the body is converted to T3. T3 is then delivered to particular organs that use predominately T3, such as the heart. Severe illness that is chronic, such as heart disease, is commonly associated with low T3 levels in the blood. This is called "low T3 syndrome." It is important to understand that the actions of T3 at the cellular level have significant affects upon the heart.

Studies have shown that it is T3 and not T4, which enters a white blood cell that then enters the blood and attacks bacteria and viruses (this cell is the cardiac monocyte). Furthermore, it is the calcium cycling proteins in the heart that are the most important target of the action of thyroid hormone. Other heart functions, such as the transport of calcium (ATPase) and the control of cardiac self-contraction, are regulated by T3. If there is not enough T3 present, then impaired diastolic function of the heart may occur. The heart muscles may not relax in a normal manner, which will result in the heart filling with blood too slowly or too quickly.

T3 also has direct effects on the mitochondria, which are rod-shaped structures that create energy and assist in the cell's function. In addition, hearts that are low in T3 show poor absorption of glucose, lactate, and free fatty acids by the mitochondria that power the heart cells. On the other hand, higher blood levels of T3 have been shown to be associated with improved heart function by increasing contractility, improved diastolic function, and lower systemic vascular resistance. Heart rate is one of the most sensitive physiological measurements of optimal thyroid function, and as it turns out, heart rate is also associated with serum T3 levels.

Consequently, medical research has shown that thyroid hormones are crucial to the daily operation of the heart. Now let's look at the effect of hypothyroidism and hyperthyroidism on heart function.

HYPOTHYROIDISM AND YOUR HEART

Many scientific studies have shown that hypothyroidism relates to an increased risk for cardiovascular disease. The heart is a major destination for thyroid hormones and any significant change in thyroid hormones will cause the heart to react.

In the hypothyroid state, thyroid hormone deficiency results in lower heart rate and weakening of myocardial contraction and relaxation, with prolonged systolic (the blood pressure when the heart is contracting) and early diastolic (the bottom number, which measures the force the heart exerts on the walls of the arteries in between beats) times, which result in altered blood pressure. Cardiac preload is decreased owing to impaired diastolic function, cardiac afterload is increased. Cardiac preload refers to the initial stretching of the cardiac muscle cells prior to when you're ready to pump out the blood in your ventricles. Cardiac afterload is the pressure against, which your heart has to contract to eject the blood. Chronotropic (alters the heart rate and rhythm by impacting the heart's electrical conduction system and the related nerves) and inotropic (impacts the contraction force of cardiac muscles) functions are reduced.

Therefore, thyroid hormone is an important regulator of cardiac function and cardiovascular hemodynamics—how your blood flows through your arteries and veins and the pressure that affects your blood flow. Triiodothyronine (T3), the physiologically active form of thyroid hormone, binds to nuclear receptor proteins and mediates the expression of several important cardiac genes. This induces transcription (copying a segment of DNA into RNA) of the positively regulated genes including alpha-myosin heavy chain (MHC) and the sarcoplasmic reticulum calcium ATPase. Negatively regulated genes include beta-MHC and phospholamban, which are down regulated in the presence of normal serum levels of thyroid hormone. T3 mediated effects on the systemic vasculature include relaxation of vascular smooth muscle resulting in decreased arterial resistance and diastolic blood pressure. In hypothyroidism, cardiac contractility and cardiac output are decreased and systemic vascular resistance (SVR) is increased.

As you probably now have surmised, thyroid hormones have numerous effects on the cardiovascular system that greatly impact heart function. Hypothyroidism is associated with the following:

- Decreased cardiac output due to impaired relaxation of vascular smooth muscle and decreased availability of endothelial nitric oxide (NO). This leads to increased arterial stiffness that leads to increased vascular resistance.

- Thyroid hormones also impact the renin-angiotensin-aldosterone system. Renin substrates are synthesized in the liver under the stimulus of T3. Thus, in a hypothyroid state, diastolic blood pressure increases, pulse pressure narrows, and renin levels decrease. This results in diastolic hypertension that is often sodium (salt) sensitive.

- Erythropoietin secretion is increased by T3, which can explain the normochromic, normocytic anemia (red blood cells are same size and have a normal red color) often found in hypothyroidism.

- Thyroid hormones also regulate pacemaker-related genes through transcription, as well as the beta-adrenergic system in cardiomyocytes—cells responsible for the contraction of the heart.

- As a result of these mechanisms, heart rate increases in the presence of thyroid hormones and decreases in hypothyroidism.

- Varied alterations in lipid parameters are noted in both overt and subclinical hypothyroidism, including elevated total cholesterol, low-density lipoprotein (LDL) cholesterol, and apolipoprotein B. A hypothyroid state results in decreased expression of hepatic LDL receptors and reduced activity of cholesterol-α-monooxygenase, which is an enzyme that breaks down cholesterol, resulting in decreased LDL clearance.

- Also noted are elevations in C-reactive protein (CRP), which is an inflammatory marker.

- Also, homocysteine levels may be elevated. High homocysteine levels increase your risk of not just heart disease and stroke, but also breast cancer, prostate cancer, memory loss, and bone loss.

- Thyroid hormones affect endothelial functions (prevent coagulation, control blood flow and passage of proteins from blood into tissues, and inhibit inflammation) mediated by thyroid hormone receptor (THR)-α_1 and THR-β. Activation of THR-α_1 increases coronary blood flow, decreases coronary resistance, and increases production of nitric oxide in endothelial and vascular smooth muscle cells. Thyroid hormone activation of THR-β induces the formation of new blood cells.

- Severe hypothyroidism can also cause pericardial effusion—buildup of fluid around the heart.

- Hypothyroidism can also be associated with a decrease in insulin sensitivity due to downregulation of glucose transporters and direct effects on insulin secretion and clearance. This phenomenon will drive up your blood sugar levels.

Signs and Symptoms

Consequently, due to the above mechanisms, individuals with low thyroid function (hypothyroidism) may have specific signs and symptoms that are related to the cardiovascular system:

- Decreased endothelial derived relaxation factor

- Decreased endurance

- Diastolic hypertension (high blood pressure)

- Elevated c-reactive protein (CRP)

- Fatigue

- Impaired cardiac contractility

- Impaired diastolic function

- Increased homocysteine (an amino acid)

- Increased serum cholesterol

- Increased systemic vascular resistance

- Mitral valve prolapse (more common in patients with Hashimoto's thyroiditis)

- Narrow pulse pressure

- Slow heart rate (bradycardia)

Hypothyroidism and Cardiovascular Complications

There are a number of specific markers that can indicate the possibility of your developing heart issues. You have a greater chance of developing cardiovascular problems if you are suffering from one or more of the following risk factors:

Atherosclerosis. People with hypothyroidism may have an increased risk of developing heart disease since they may have a higher rate of hardening of the arteries (atherosclerosis). Trials have also shown an increase in abdominal aortic atherosclerosis in patients with mild hypothyroidism.

Cardiac fibroblasts. Hypothyroidism may promote an abnormal thickening of the heart valves (myocardial fibrosis) by stimulating fibroblasts, which is the opposite of, which occurs in hyperthyroidism. Cardiac fibroblasts are the largest cell group in the heart, and they contribute to the structural, biochemical, mechanical, and electrical properties of the myocardium (the muscular tissue of the heart).

Cholesterol. One study showed a direct relationship between the level of TSH and serum total cholesterol and LDL (bad cholesterol). High cholesterol can be affected by your thyroid, and it can alter your heart health. Furthermore, it can lead to strokes since plaque can build up in your arteries elsewhere in your body. Studies have also shown that in hypothyroid individuals, LDL (blood cholesterol) may rise.

Creatine kinase. Trials have also shown that serum creatine kinase (an enzyme found in the heart) is elevated by 50 percent in about 30 percent of patients with hypothyroidism. An elevated level of creatine kinase is seen within hours of a heart attack when the heart muscle is damaged. Also, fluid around the heart (pericardial effusions) may occur due to the increase in volume of distribution of albumin and the decrease in lymphatic clearance that may occur commonly in patients with hypothyroidism.

Low T3 levels. Trials in both humans and animals have shown that low thyroid hormone levels contribute to a poorer outcome after acute myocardial infarction (heart attack). A rapid decline in free T3 was found during the first week after a heart attack. Reverse T3 also was increased, but free T4 remained normal. Another study showed that in-hospital and post-discharge death rate was higher among individuals with lower T3 levels and higher reverse T3 levels.

Statin drugs. Some people have difficulty taking statin drugs to lower their cholesterol since the medications in some individuals are associated with the development of a cardiac myopathy (a muscular disease). This myopathy has been associated with low coenzyme Q-10 levels. It has also been shown that the myopathy that can be caused by statin drugs may be associated with mild thyroid insufficiency. Consequently, all patients taking a statin drug should be evaluated for hypothyroidism and treated if appropriate.

Diagnosis and Treatment

The first step in determining if you may be suffering from heart disease is getting a doctor's physical exam. Your healthcare provider will then decide, which test to administer in order to make a diagnosis.

Echocardiogram

An echocardiogram (ECHO) is an ultrasound that measures how electrical impulses move through heart muscle allowing your doctor to view your heart beating and pumping blood. The echocardiogram shows mild to moderate large pericardial effusions in up to 30 percent of people with severe hypothyroidism. The pericardial output however is usually not decreased. When the individual is prescribed thyroid hormone the fluid around the heart usually resolves in a few weeks to a few months.

Electrocardiogram

An electrocardiogram (EKG) is a static picture of the heart used to assess your heart rhythm, to measure the heart flow to the heart, to diagnose an enlarged heart, and to diagnose a heart attack. The EKG changes in patients with hypothyroidism may include any of the following:

- Lengthened duration of contraction, which predisposes people to ventricular arrhythmias (irregular heart rhythms)

- Low voltage

- Sinus bradycardia (slower than average heart rate)

SUBCLINICAL HYPOTHYROIDISM

Subclinical (undetected) hypothyroidism is categorized as a mild to moderate form of hypothyroidism. It is an early phase of the disease, and it has no, or few, clinical symptoms that are detectable. Individuals with subclinical hypothyroidism are usually people with elevated TSH levels but have normal serum free or total T4 and normal free T3. The incidence of subclinical hypothyroidism increases with age. In younger patients it is more common in women. In older people the rate is evenly split between men and women. The reported prevalence of subclinical hypothyroidism depends on several factors, such as iodine supplementation, age, and race. In the United States, the prevalence of subclinical hypothyroidism is reported as 4.3 percent in the NHANES III study and as high as 9.5 percent in the Colorado study. The annual risk of progression to overt hypothyroidism is reported at 1 percent to 5 percent, depending on TSH levels and thyroid antibody status. Patients with subclinical hypothyroidism manifest many of the same cardiovascular changes, but commonly to a lesser degree than that, which occurs in overt hypothyroidism. However, as described earlier, cardiovascular changes of arterial compliance, diastolic blood pressure, endothelial dysfunction, and hyperlipidemia that are noted with overt hypothyroidism can also occur in subclinical hypothyroidism.

A study conducted in individuals with subclinical hypothyroidism, dyslipidemia (high cholesterol) was shown to be common. Furthermore, as abnormal cholesterol levels rose, the higher the TSH value. The authors concluded that subclinical hypothyroidism needs to be treated to prevent the complications of dyslipidemia, which is an atherogenic condition as it increases overall cardiovascular risk. Another study revealed that subclinical hypothyroidism was associated with a significantly higher LDL (bad cholesterol) and lower HDL (good cholesterol) levels than the control group regardless of the age of the participants. Yet another study showed that patients with subclinical hypothyroidism had significantly higher total cholesterol, triglycerides, and LDL-C levels, as well as significantly lower levels of HDL-C in comparison to the healthy controls. In general, subclinical hypothyroidism increases the risk of cardiovascular heart disease (CHD) mortality, and CHD events, but not of total mortality (death from any cause). Several of those and other studies suggested an increased risk of coronary heart disease and cardiovascular mortality in younger individuals with the cut-off age varying from 50 to 70 years. Moreover, several trials have shown a strong link between subclinical hypothyroidism and poor outcome in people with and without heart disease. In patients with chronic heart failure, TSH levels that are even slightly above normal are found to be independently associated with an increased risk of progression of heart failure. This is one of the reasons that it is important to treat subclinical hypothyroidism.

In addition, there are changes that may occur in thyroid metabolism in patients with heart disease. Interestingly, an alteration may occur in the metabolism of thyroid hormone if the patient has heart disease, has had heart surgery, or has had a heart attack. Commonly you may have a low free T3 with normal TSH and free T4 levels. This is called low-T3 syndrome.

Low-T3 Syndrome

Low-T3 syndrome is a strong predictor of death in cardiac patients and might be directly implicated in the poor prognosis of cardiac patients. Furthermore, in people with heart failure, there is commonly a decrease in serum T3 concentration, which is usually proportional to the severity of the disease. In addition, if the person has a low ratio of T3 to reverse T3, it is a predictor of increased mortality if the individual has congestive heart failure.

Studies have shown that if the individual is given T3 then the cardiac output is increased, and the systemic vascular resistance is decreased, and they improve. An abnormal heart rhythm (ventricular tachycardia) has been shown to be associated with low T3 or low T3/T4 ratio and increased levels of reverse T3. In fact, one study showed that elevated reverse T3 levels was the strongest predictor of mortality in the first year after having a heart attack. Also, low T3 has also been shown to be predictive of developing an abnormal heart rhythm (atrial fibrillation) after having open heart surgery. Furthermore, low T3 levels are a predictor of an increase in death rate in patients with heart disease. Another study showed that thyroid hormone dysfunction plays an important role in the progression to dilated cardiomyopathy, which is a syndrome where the heart gets larger and eventually fails. When the subjects in the study were given thyroid hormone replacement, they had significant improvement.

Again, it is very important that you have optimal thyroid function in many aspects, but particularly when it comes to the prevention and treatment of heart disease. Women with TSH levels in the upper reference range have increased arterial stiffness compared to women with lower TSH. This increases their risk of heart disease. This study was done on postmenopausal women. T3 is also important in the regulation of cardiac gene expression. Furthermore, the list of T3-mediated genes that are changed in hypothyroidism are very similar to the changes in gene expression in heart failure.

Signs and Symptoms

If your physician believes that you may be suffering from subclinical hypothyroidism because you may be experiencing mild symptoms, such as fatigue, depression, consistent weight gain, or memory problems, he/she may order lab tests to support the diagnosis. If you are diagnosed with subclinical hypothyroidism, it should be monitored and treated to achieve optimal thyroid function and to decrease the risk of heart disease. Other signs and symptoms of subclinical hypothyroidism that are related to the cardiovascular system are:

- Cholesterol levels increase parallel with an increase in TSH levels about 5 mU/L.

- Independent risk factor for atherosclerosis and heart attack in females.

- Higher rate of hardening of the arteries, altered cardiac contractility, and systemic vascular resistance.

- Positive thyroid antibodies increase the risk of acute myocardial infarction.

Treatment

Research has shown and recommended that, from a cardiac perspective, individuals with subclinical hypothyroidism be treated with thyroid hormone. A medical trial of patients with subclinical hypothyroidism showed benefits on cardiovascular risk factors and quality of life when they were supplemented with thyroid hormone. Another study also showed that after thyroid hormone replacement lipid (cholesterol) levels improved, resistance to pumping blood (systemic vascular resistance) lowered, and the ability of heart self-contraction (heart contractility) was also enhanced.

Moreover, one study showed that heart disease mortality in female patients and also abnormal serum lipids for people were more common if they had subclinical hypothyroidism. Last, a study done using the United Kingdom General Practitioner research database revealed an important finding. It found that 53 percent of people who were under the age of 70 that were treated with levothyroxine for their subclinical hypothyroidism, had a reduction in recurring chest pain or discomfort (ischemic heart disease events), as well as death from cardiovascular disease.

Low T3 syndrome has been found to be a strong prognostic, independent predictor of death in people with acute and chronic heart disease.

Likewise, individuals with heart disease that have normal thyroid function were found to have lower levels of T3 compared to healthy patients. Consequently, it is imperative that when your doctor evaluates thyroid function, if you have subclinical hypothyroidism, optimal levels of thyroid hormone be achieved and that T3 also be replaced along with T4. One study found that alterations in gene expression are reversible after restoring normal T3 plasma levels by giving T3. Moreover, it is paramount to note that there is no significant intracellular deiodinase activity in cardiac cells; therefore, the heart relies mainly on the action of T3 since that is the hormone transported into the myocyte (muscle cell in the heart).

OTHER MARKERS FOR INCREASED RISK OF HEART DISEASE ASSOCIATED WITH HYPOTHYROIDISM

Thyroid gland disorders can directly change the normal role of the heart causing symptoms and resulting in serious complications. Additional key indicators for increased risk of heart disease are elevated levels of C-reactive protein (CRP) and homocysteine in the blood. These markers can also be linked to hypothyroidism. Another risk factor for heart disease that is related to hypothyroidism that is not discussed commonly is apolipoprotein-B. As you are about to see, improving an underactive thyroid condition can also improve your cardiovascular health by improving other cardiac markers.

C-reactive Protein (CRP)

C-reactive protein is a marker for inflammation in the body and if elevated is a major risk factor for cardiovascular disease. CRP is produced in the liver, and it is measured by administering a blood test. Elevated levels occur when there is inflammation in the lining of the arteries, which leads to the formation of plaque and eventually a narrowing of the walls of the blood vessels.

Causes of Elevated Levels

Elevated levels of CRP are caused by infection and many long-term conditions, such as cancer, lupus, pain resulting from swelling of the blood vessels (giant cell arteritis), rheumatoid arthritis, infection of the bone (osteomyelitis), rheumatic fever, tuberculosis, and inflammatory bowel syndrome. Elevated levels of CRP are also seen in some patients at menopause and also in some women with polycystic ovarian syndrome (PCOS). High levels of CRP may furthermore be a risk factor for diabetes and hypertension. When evaluating the patient for heart disease, commonly your doctor will order a special kind of C-reactive protein test called high-sensitivity CRP (hs-CRP). High-sensitivity C-reactive protein is a marker of inflammation that predicts incident myocardial infarction, stroke, peripheral arterial disease, and sudden cardiac death among healthy individuals with no history of cardiovascular disease, and recurrent events and death in patients with acute or stable coronary syndromes. Hs-CRP confers additional prognostic value at all levels of cholesterol, Framingham coronary risk score, severity of the metabolic syndrome, and blood pressure, and in those with and without subclinical atherosclerosis.

Test Results

The following are recommendations made by the American Heart Association in relation to cardiovascular risk and CRP levels:

- 1 mg per liter or lower is regarded as low risk

- 1 to 3 mg per liter is regarded as moderate risk

- 3 mg or greater is regarded as high risk

- levels higher than 1mg per liter may indicate a heart attack or a great risk of having a myocardial infarction

Treatment

You can lower your CRP level with natural foods, diet, vitamins, omega-3 fatty acids, herbs, and supplements. Specifically, the following are ways to lower C-reactive protein:

- Antibiotics (if an infection is present or levels are very elevated)

- Baby aspirin, one per day (check with your doctor first)

- Balancing hormones in women with PCOS

- Coenzyme Q-10

- Curcumin (200 to 600 mg a day)

- Essential fatty acids such as fish oil or EPA/DHA (1,000 mg a day)

- Grapeseed extract (100 to 200 mg per day)

- Green tea (3 cups per day)

- Low-dose naltrexone (LDN)

- Moderate exercise

- Natural estrogen replacement in menopausal women that are deficient and are able to take estrogen

- Quercetin supplementation or foods or drinks high in quercetin, such as apples and onions or black tea

- Rosemary

- Statin drugs that are used to lower cholesterol

- Thyroid medication if you are hypothyroid

Homocysteine

Homocysteine levels are commonly elevated in people with hypothyroidism. Homocysteine is an amino acid. High levels in the body induce endothelial dysfunction and lead to atherogenic (promotes formation of fatty plaques in the arteries) changes in the lipid profile. This process is also one of the causes of oxidative stress, which can lead to vascular disease and heart disease.

Oxidative stress is a term used to describe internal inflammation and the free radicals produced as a result of this inflammation. High homocysteine levels can damage the arterial lining of the heart, making it narrow and inelastic, a condition also known as "hardening" of the arteries (arteriosclerosis). When levels are elevated, homocysteine can also reduce nitric oxide production, which can lead to high blood pressure, which is also a risk factor for heart disease. Furthermore, some researchers believe that high homocysteine levels also increase the risk of blood clotting, which decreases blood flow through the arteries. One study showed that women with a history of high blood pressure and elevated homocysteine levels were twenty-five times more likely to have a heart attack or stroke than women whose blood pressure and homocysteine levels were closer to normal.

Last, if homocysteine levels are high this is usually reflective of decreased methylation in the body, which increases your risk of not only heart disease but other diseases as well.

Causes of Elevated Levels

The following are causes of high homocysteine:

- Hereditary predisposition related to poor methylation

- Hypothyroidism

- Medications

- Menopause

- Nutritional deficiencies of vitamins B_6, B_{12}, and folate

- PCOS

- Renal failure

- Smoking

- Toxins

In incidences where high homocysteine levels are hereditary, it is may be due to the fact that some people are lacking the enzyme methyl tetra-hydrofolate reductase, which breaks down homocysteine. This enzyme is an important part of the methylation pathway. A deficiency of this enzyme increases the need for a special type of folate (folic acid) in order to prevent high homocysteine levels. This occurs in at least 12 percent of the population of the United States. High homocysteine levels have been found to be associated with an increased risk in not just heart disease and stroke, but also osteoporosis, depression, memory loss, multiple sclerosis, type II diabetes, renal (kidney) failure, depression, rheumatoid arthritis, and prostate and breast cancer.

Test Results

An optimal level of homocysteine is 6 to 8 micromoles/liter. Anything outside of this range should be addressed. Low levels can be just as dangerous as high levels.

Treatment

The following are ways to lower homocysteine levels:

- Exercise

- Increasing intake of broccoli, spinach, Brussels sprouts, cabbage, Bok choy, or cauliflower (remember from Chapter 2 that too many of these vegetables can decrease the conversion of T4 to T3 and then negatively affect thyroid function, therefore use in moderation)

- Natural estrogen replacement therapy placed on the skin, in patients that have low estrogen and are candidates for natural prescription estrogen replacement

- SAMe (s-adenosylmethionine), 200 to 400 mg a day

- Stress reduction

- Supplementation with vitamins B_6, B_{12}, folate or the activated form of folate, methyltetrahydrofolate, the activated form of B_6, which is pyridoxal-5-phosphate, and the activated form of B_{12}, which is methylcobalamin

- TMG (trimethylglycine) 400 to 500 mg twice a day

Amazingly, researchers have suggested that folate supplementation could save 20,000 to 50,000 lives from heart disease every year.

Apolipoprotein-B (apoB)

Cholesterol-rich, apolipoprotein B (apoB)-containing lipoproteins are now widely accepted as the most important causal agents of atherosclerotic cardiovascular disease. Apolipoprotein-B, the critical structural protein of the atherogenic lipoproteins, has two major isoforms: apoB48 and apoB100. Apolipoprotein B-48 (apoB-48) is a major apolipoprotein of intestine-derived chylomicrons—triglyceride-rich lipoproteins—(CM) and CM remnants (CMR). ApoB levels indicate the atherogenic particle concentration independent of the particle cholesterol content, which is variable. While LDL, the major cholesterol-carrying serum lipoprotein, is the primary therapeutic target for management and prevention of atherosclerotic cardiovascular disease, there is strong evidence that apoB is a more accurate indicator of cardiovascular risk than either total cholesterol or LDL cholesterol. Studies have shown that thyroid function influences serum apolipoprotein B-48 levels in patients with hypothyroidism.

HYPERTHYROIDISM AND YOUR HEART

Hyperthyroidism can also lead to complications in the body. It can directly alter the normal workings of the heart and vascular system causing serious complications. For patients with an overactive thyroid as seen in hyperthyroidism, existing cardiac symptoms can worsen or it can cause new ones in healthy hearts. Overall, hyperthyroidism is characterized by an increase in resting heart rate, blood volume, stroke volume (the volume of blood pumped from the left ventricle per beat), myocardial contractility, and ejection fraction.

Hemodynamic changes (blood flow through the arteries and veins and forces affecting blood flow) in hyperthyroidism are related to the role of catecholamines—hormones made by adrenal glands—and the role of renin-angiotensin-aldosterone system (RAAS)—regulates blood volume, electrolytes, and systemic vascular resistance (SVR). In the RAAS system, preload is increased in a state of hyperthyroidism, and the reduced peripheral vascular resistance and elevated heart rate lead to increased cardiac output. The reduction in systemic vascular resistance results in decreased renal (kidney) perfusion pressure and activation of the renin-angiotensin-aldosterone system, thereby increasing sodium reabsorption and blood volume. In turn, this leads to increased preload, decreased afterload, and ultimately a significant increase in stroke volume. In addition, there is evidence that T3 directly stimulates the synthesis of renin substrate in the liver and enhances the cardiac expression of renin mRNA, leading to increased cardiac levels of renin (an enzyme secreted by kidneys to regulate blood pressure) and angiotensin II (higher than normal angiotensin II levels cause excess fluid retention and high blood pressure) that are independent of the circulating renin and angiotensin (a peptide hormone that regulates blood pressure). Therefore, it is essential that this thyroid condition be identified and treated correctly in order to prevent heart disease or to decrease cardiovascular symptoms. (See Chapter 4 on page 75 for more details on hyperthyroidism.)

Heart Failure In Hyperthyroidism

The development of "high-output heart failure" in hyperthyroidism may be due to "tachycardia-mediated cardiomyopathy," which is a reversible ventricular dysfunction and leads to heart failure. More specifically, thy-rotoxic cardiomyopathy is defined as myocardial damage caused by toxic effects of excessive thyroid hormone, resulting in altered myocyte energy production, intracellular metabolism, and myofibril contractile function (produces muscle contraction and relaxation). The main manifestations are left ventricular hypertrophy (thickening of the walls of the lower left heart chamber), heart rhythm disturbances, primary atrial fibrillation, dilation of the heart chambers, heart failure, pulmonary hypertension, and diastolic dysfunction (problem with diastole the first part of your heartbeat).

Patients with high-output heart failure can manifest with symptoms such as dyspnea (difficulty breathing) on exertion, fatigue, and fluid retention with peripheral edema (too much fluid in the lungs), pleural effusion (an unusual amount of fluid around the lung), hepatic (liver) congestion, and pulmonary hypertension. An untreated high-output state and hyperthyroidism can lead to ventricular dilation, persistent tachycardia (increased heart rate), and eventual chronic heart failure (failure of the heart to pump effectively) that can result in a fatal event. In a study by Mitchell et al., heart failure patients with abnormal thyroid function had a 60 percent higher risk of mortality compared to individuals with normal thyroid function with heart failure.

Signs and Symptoms

There are many cardiovascular symptoms of hyperthyroidism that you should be aware of, such as the following:

- Chest pain related to the heart (angina)
- Exercise intolerance
- High blood pressure (systolic hypertension)
- Increased cardiac output
- Irregular heartbeat (atrial fibrillation)
- Palpitations, increased heart rate (tachycardia)
- Pulmonary hypertension
- Shortness of breath
- Swelling of the extremities (edema)
- Wide pulse pressure due to the increase in systolic and decease in diastolic pressure due to reduced resistance, lower resistance is due to an increase in nitric oxide production

HYPERTHYROIDISM AND CARDIOVASCULAR COMPLICATIONS

If hyperthyroidism is left untreated, it can lead to other health problems, such as cardiovascular or heart issues. The following are specific heart signs that your physician may find if you have hyperthyroidism.

Cardiac hypertrophy. When your heart has to pump harder in order to deliver blood to the rest of your body it may result in an enlarged heart. An enlarged heart may be associated with an overactive thyroid.

Congestive Heart Failure. When your heart is not able to pump blood to the organs of the body adequately and meet the demands placed on it, you may be suffering from congestive heart failure. In many cases alterations in thyroid hormone metabolism accompanies congestive heart failure. Congestive heart failure usually occurs in individuals that already have underlying heart disease and not as much in people that were young and healthy before they developed hyperthyroidism.

Inotropic effect. An inotropic effect can be applied to the conditions that alter the force of muscular contraction. Thyroid hormone production in excessive amounts has a direct inotropic effect on the heart muscle and cardiac contraction.

Irregular Heart Sounds. Irregular heart sounds may be enhanced and a scratchy systolic sound along the left sternal border may be present. When normal metabolic rate is restored, the symptoms and signs usually resolve.

Mitral Valve Prolapse. Mitral valve prolapse is a condition in, which the two valve flaps of the mitral valve, during contraction, do not close evenly. This condition may result in a heart murmur. Mitral valve prolapse occurs more commonly in Graves' disease or Hashimoto's thyroiditis than in the general population.

Peripheral Resistance. Peripheral resistance (systemic vascular resistance SVR) is the exertion against the blood flow in the body. When the patient is at rest, the peripheral resistance is decreased, and the cardiac output is increased. Hyperthyroidism results in a high output of the thyroid hormone and this hormone induced effect decreases the total peripheral resistance. The heart reacts to the low peripheral resistance by increasing the heart rate. If left untreated an elevation in heart rate can increase the risk of developing a stroke.

Systolic and Diastolic Pressure. Your blood pressure readings are an indication of the amount of force or pressure that blood exerts on the blood vessels as it moves through. The systolic number (top) measures the amount of pressure the blood wields while the heart is beating. The diastolic number (bottom) measures the pressure in your vessels between heartbeats. These numbers can be affected by your hormone levels. An overactive thyroid can lead to high systolic blood pressure.

Hyperthyroidism in People Over 60

Irregular heart rhythm (atrial fibrillation) occurs in 10 to 15 percent of hyperthyroid patients, of which most are 60 and older. Restoring normal heart rhythm is necessary since they are at an increased risk for blood clots (thromboembolic events), particularly if they already have a history of heart disease, high blood pressure, or previous blood clots or pulmonary embolism, which is a blood clot that blocks blood flow to an artery in the lung.

Likewise, subclinical hyperthyroidism often manifests itself differently in elderly patients. Older patients with subclinical hyperthyroidism are also at increased risk of developing atrial fibrillation. The following are potential heart problems associated with subclinical hyperthyroidism in the elderly.

- Decreased large and small artery elasticity

- Impaired left ventricular diastolic filling

- Impaired systolic function during exercise

- Increased cardiac contractility

- Increased intraventricular septal thickness

- Increased left ventricular mass index

- Increased left ventricular posterior wall thickness

- Prolonged QT interval

Also, long-term studies of older people with untreated subclinical hyperthyroidism showed an increased risk of developing heart disease and death from all causes. Therefore, it is imperative that subclinical hyperthyroidism be treated. Treatment has been shown to improve the following cardiac functions:

- Decrease in atrial and ventricular premature beats

- Decrease in heart rate

- Decrease in left ventricular posterior wall thickness at diastole

- Reduction in interventricular septum thickness

- Reduction in left ventricular mass index

Heart (cardiac) output may be increased as much as 50 to 300 percent due to the combined effect of increased resting heart rate, increased contractility, increased flow of blood, increased blood volume, and decreased resistance the blood experiences as it circulates throughout the body (systemic vascular resistance). It is interesting that the cardiovascular symptoms and signs are independent of the cause of the hyperthyroidism. In individuals that have pulmonary hypertension and hyperthyroidism, it may be associated with right-sided heart failure. The symptoms are due to increased circulatory demands from hyper-metabolism and the need for the body to decrease the excess heat produced. These complications are generally reversible with appropriate treatment.

Sinus Tachycardia and Atrial Fibrillation. Sinus tachycardia (heart beats faster than normal at rest) is the most common rhythm disturbance and is recorded in almost all patients with hyperthyroidism. Therefore, an increase in resting heart rate is characteristic of this disease. However, it is atrial fibrillation that is most commonly identified with thyrotoxicosis. The prevalence of atrial fibrillation in this disease ranges between 2 percent and 20 percent. When compared with a control population with normal thyroid function, a prevalence of atrial fibrillation of 2.3 percent stands in contrast to 13.8 percent in patients with overt hyperthyroidism.

Subclinical Hyperthyroidism and the Heart

Subclinical hyperthyroidism is characterized by a low or undetectable serum TSH concentration in the presence of normal levels of serum T_4 and T_3. Patients may have no clinical signs or symptoms; however, studies show that they are at risk for many of the cardiovascular manifestations associated with overt hyperthyroidism. The risk of CHD mortality and atrial fibrillation (but not other outcomes) in subclinical hyperthyroidism is higher among patients with very low levels of thyrotropin (TSH).

TREATMENT

Therapies for hyperthyroidism depend on the cause and severity of the symptoms. Treatment of the hyperthyroidism usually returns cardiac function to normal. Treatment of atrial fibrillation in the setting of hyperthyroidism includes beta-adrenergic blockade (taking a beta blocker). Rapid diagnosis of hyperthyroidism and successful treatment with either radioiodine or thioureas is associated with a reversion to sinus rhythm in a majority of patients within 2 to 3 months. In fact, 60 percent of people who have atrial fibrillation convert without cardio conversion (a medical procedure slowing down a fast heart rate to a normal heart rate) to normal heart rhythm after they are treated for their hyperthyroidism within four months. Consequently, younger people are not usually given a blood thinner if they have no history of underlying heart disease or history of a prior problem with blood clots. If the person does not convert their heart rhythm to a normal one by taking medication to improve their heart rhythm, then cardio conversion is usually very successful up to one year after the diagnosis of thyrotoxicosis. Older patients (>60 years old) with atrial fibrillation of longer duration are less likely to spontaneously revert to sinus rhythm. Therefore, after the patient has been rendered chemically euthyroid, if atrial fibrillation persists, electrical or pharmacological cardioversion may be attempted.

AMIODARONE-INDUCED THYROID DYSFUNCTION

Amiodarone is a highly effective antiarrhythmic drug used for the treatment of both atrial and ventricular cardiac rhythm disturbances. Amiodarone inhibits the conversion of T4 to T3 due to the inhibition of 5'-deiodinase activity. It is 37 percent iodine by weight and has a half-life of one hundred days. Secondary to its iodine content and chemical structure, which is similar to thyroid hormone, it may cause thyroid abnormalities. The risk is greater if you have positive thyroid antibodies. Amiodarone-induced hypothyroidism (AIT) occurs in 5 percent to 10 percent of treated patients and is more common in iodine-sufficient areas of the world. At first, TSH levels may be normal then the individual may become hypothyroid.

Amiodarone may also cause hyperthyroidism. It occurs in 2 percent to 10 percent of treated individuals. Amiodarone-induced hyperthyroidism is more frequently found in iodine-deficient areas of the world. First symptoms of amiodarone-induced thyrotoxicosis may be a new onset or recurrence of ventricular irritability (irritability of the heart), return or worsening heart failure symptoms and/or changes in Coumadin (a blood thinner) dose requirements. Thyrotoxicosis induced by amiodarone has two forms:

- Type I AIT is more common in iodine-deficient areas and is associated with preexisting thyroid abnormalities such as autonomous nodular goiter or Graves' disease

- Type II AIT is the result of amiodarone causing a subacute thyroiditis with release of preformed thyroid hormones into the circulation

CONCLUSION

As you have seen in this chapter, there is an important relationship between a well-functioning thyroid gland and the state of your cardio-vascular health—a relationship, which gets more important as you grow older. Understanding what happens to your heart when your thyroid malfunctions can be a matter of life and death. By being aware of the signs, by having an annual check-up, and asking the right questions, you can add years to your life. Knowing what to do when your thyroid malfunctions is key. Since the heart is very vulnerable to a reduction in free T3, when thyroid medication is needed, thyroid hormone replacement therapy with a combination of T3 and T4 has been found to be helpful to prevent and treat heart disease. If you have hyperthyroidism, reducing thyroid hormone output is paramount to help your heart return to health-ier function. Hopefully, the information in this chapter will provide you with the options you may be searching for.

10

Thyroid Hormones and Hypertension

Both hypothyroidism and hyperthyroidism have been associated with hypertension (high blood pressure).

Blood pressure is the measurement of the blood's force in the arteries as the heart pushes the blood through the body. High blood pressure occurs when too much pressure is exerted on the artery walls by the blood. A blood pressure reading consists of two numbers: systolic and diastolic. Systolic blood pressure is the top number and refers to the amount of pressure experienced by the arteries while the heart is beating. Diastolic blood pressure is the bottom number and refers to the amount of pressure in the arteries while the heart is resting in between heartbeats.

While some people with early-stage hypertension experience dull headaches, dizziness, or nosebleeds, most sufferers have no symptoms whatsoever. Nevertheless, when untreated, high blood pressure increases your risk for heart disease, stroke, kidney disease, and congestive heart failure. This is why it is sometimes referred to as the "silent killer."

Globally, high blood pressure is the leading risk factor for cardiovascular disease morbidity and mortality. About 75 million American adults (29 percent) have high blood pressure, which is 1 in every 3 American adults. The new American College of Cardiology/American Heart Association guidelines eliminate the classification of *prehypertension* and divides it into two levels: (1) elevated BP, with a systolic pressure (SBP) between 120 and 129 mm Hg and diastolic pressure (DBP) less than 80 mm Hg, and (2) stage 1 hypertension, with an SBP of 130 to 139 mm Hg or a DBP of 80 to 89 mm Hg. The current definition of hypertension (HTN) is systolic blood pressure (SBP) values of 130 or more and/or diastolic blood pressure (DBP) more than 80 mm Hg.

Hypertension can cause significant morbidity and reduced life expectancy. Most people with hypertension have primary (essential) hypertension where there is the absence of an identifiable secondary cause; however, 10 to 15 percent of patients have secondary hypertension. Secondary hypertension is when there is an identifiable, and potentially reversible, cause of your hypertension. Endocrine disorders explain approximately 10 percent of secondary hypertension and thyroid disorders account for approximately 1 percent of those cases.

Hypothyroidism

If you have subclinical hypothyroidism, you are at a higher risk of developing hypertension and dyslipidemia where total cholesterol and LDL cholesterol levels are elevated. In other words, hypothyroidism has been recognized as a cause of secondary hypertension. Increased peripheral vascular resistance and low cardiac output has been suggested to be the possible link between hypothyroidism and diastolic hypertension. In addition, an inflammatory response is commonly initiated with the individual developing elevated levels of c-reactive protein and IL-6, which are inflammatory markers.

Furthermore, endothelial dysfunction may occur due to low levels of nitric oxide (NO). Endothelial dysfunction is a type of coronary artery disease, which is due to a lack of nitric oxide inside of your blood vessel walls that cause the arteries to narrow. Moreover, the hypothyroid population is characterized by significant volume changes, which initiates a volume-dependent, low plasma renin activity mechanism of blood pressure elevation. There is also an increase in plaque formation as well as arterial stiffness. The good news is that hypertension may be reversible in 50 percent of patients by hormone replacement therapy with thyroid hormone if the patient is hypothyroid.

Hyperthyroidism

Hyperthyroidism can cause increased cardiac output, increased systolic blood pressures, and increased levels of renin, angiotensin, and aldosterone. In hyperthyroidism, elevation of diastolic blood pressure is uncommon. Systolic hypertension is more common in younger age groups. An increase in cardiac output and a decrease in total peripheral resistance accompany the hyperthyroidism. Potentiation of catecholamine action (narrowing blood vessels and raising your heart rate) by an excess of thyroid hormone has been invoked as an explanation, because thyroid hormone excess is accompanied by increased beta-adrenergic receptors in some tissue, including the heart. Treatment of the hyperthyroidism lowers systolic blood pressure in most patients and may cure hypertension in some people. Consequently, identifying secondary hypertension has important benefits.

TREATMENT OF HIGH BLOOD PRESSURE (HYPERTENSION)

Lifestyle changes are very important to decrease your risk of developing hypertension and to treat it if it begins. The Dietary Approaches to Stop Hypertension (DASH) diet, Mediterranean diet, vegetarian diet, and raw foods have all been shown to be beneficial to lower blood pressure. There are also some foods that have been shown to reduce blood pressure, such as bananas, onions, leafy greens, red beets, whole oats, garlic, soy, flaxseed, and pomegranate juice. Using sesame oil as your cooking oil may also lower your blood pressure according to a medical study. In addition, studies reveal that the consumption of 2.5 grams a day of unsweetened cocoa powder, which is rich in flavanols, lowers blood pressure in individuals that already have hypertension. Moreover, beetroot contains high levels of dietary nitrate (NO_3), which the body converts into biologically active nitrite (NO_2) and nitric oxide (NO). In the human body, NO relaxes and dilates blood vessels. Studies have shown that beetroot juice/chews lower blood pressure.

Although medications can reduce blood pressure to normal levels, they can also have a range of side effects, including depression; constipation; dizziness; fatigue; deficiencies of potassium, magnesium, and other nutrients; kidney damage; impaired sexual function; and decreased alertness and memory. Fortunately, certain supplements can help you lower your blood pressure without the use of drugs. (See the table below.) Other supplements can be used with drugs to augment their effects. Just keep in mind that hypertension is a serious disorder, so whether you are using these supplements to minimize or eventually discontinue your use of antihypertensive drugs, you must work with a physician to make sure that your blood pressure is being properly controlled. If you are currently taking blood pressure medication, do not stop taking it without the approval of your doctor. It is also critical to recognize that a good diet and regular exercise are extremely important in lowering and then maintaining your blood pressure. In addition, stress-reducing techniques such as prayer,

Risk Factors for High Blood Pressure

Although scientists don't know exactly why some people have high blood pressure and some do not, they have identified a number of risk factors for high blood pressure. The following are some of the factors associated with hypertension.

- Age (being over 55)

- Alcohol abuse

- Excess weight

- Genetics

- Lack of exercise

- Poor diet--especially one that is high in sodium, saturated fat, trans fatty acids, sugar, refined carbohydrates, and caffeine

- Smoking

- Stress

- Use of certain drugs, including amphetamine-like medications; cocaine; steroids; cyclosporine; decongestants; ephedra; erythropoietin; certain antidepressants; nonsteroidal anti-inflammatory drugs (NSAIDs), such as aspirin; COX inhibitors; and birth control and estrogen replacement pills

medication, tai chi, yoga, exercise, and breathing techniques can further help you lower your blood pressure.

Your doctor may feel that it is necessary for you to take one of the following types of medications. Yet, as stated above, many blood pressure medications cause a wide range of side effects. There are often nutrients that can be taken to augment the effects of the medication, so that a lower dosage can be used. This often causes many of the negative effects to subside. You may even find that the nutrient can replace the medication. Before taking any nutrients on the following lists, however, discuss your options with your healthcare provider.

Diuretics

Diuretics can lower your blood pressure quite effectively. Unfortunately, they can also increase your risk of other health problems. The following

TABLE 10.1. SUPPLEMENTS THAT CAN LOWER BLOOD PRESSURE

Supplements	Dosage	Considerations
Alpha lipoic acid	300 mg once a day	Alpha lipoic acid can interact with medication taken for diabetes and thyroid problems. Speak to your healthcare provider to see if any of the medications you take make it unwise to use this supplement.
Arginine	2,000 mg three times a day	Do not take if you have kidney disease, liver disease, or herpes except under a doctor's supervision. Arginine can interact with some medications. Consult with your healthcare provider before beginning this therapy.
B-complex vitamins	50 mg twice a day	I suggest taking a multivitamin along with your B-complex vitamins.
Calcium	500 mg twice a day	Although most people are deficient in calcium, there is a danger in taking too much. Do not ingest more than 1,000 to 1,200 mg of calcium a day.
Carnitine*	1,000 to 2,000 mg once a day	Have your healthcare provider measure your TMAO levels before starting long-term supplementation.
Cocoa	2.5 g (0.1 ounce) unsweetened cocoa powder (about 0.5 teaspoon)	Cocoa can interact with some medications, so speak to your healthcare provider or pharmacist before starting long-term supplementation. Be aware that cocoa contains caffeine.
Coenzyme Q-10*	60 to 120 mg once a day	If you are on blood-thinning medications, speak to your healthcare provider before using CoQ-10. Since some medications can cause a deficiency of this nutrient, speak to your healthcare provider to determine if you might need a larger dose.
Cysteine	1,000 mg once a day as n-acetylcysteine, or NAC	When taking NAC supplements, also take extra vitamin C, copper, and zinc.
EPA/DHA (fish oil)*	3,000 to 4,000 mg once a day	Choose a source that contains vitamin E to prevent oxidation. In high doses, fatty acids may cause the blood to thin. If you are taking a blood thinner, do not take EPA/DHA without direct instructions from your doctor. It is important to maintain the proper ratio of omega-6 fatty acids to omega-3 fatty acids.
Garlic*	10 mg allicin or a total allicin potential of 4,000 mcg (equal to one clove of garlic) once a day	Garlic is a blood thinner. Do not use if you are taking any kind of blood-thinning medication or supplements.

Supplements	Dosage	Considerations
Hawthorn*	160 to 900 mg of dried standardized extract once a day	Hawthorn can interact with a number of medications. Speak to your healthcare provider or pharmacist to learn if any drugs you're taking might make it unwise to take hawthorn.
Lycopene	10 to 20 mg once a day	May cause GI problems such as diarrhea and gas.
Magnesium	600 to 800 mg once a day	Consult your healthcare provider for dosage if you have kidney disease. Discontinue use and see your doctor if you experience abdominal pain. Take a lower dose if it causes diarrhea.
Potassium	See your healthcare provider for dosage directions.	
Quercetin*	50 mg three times a day	For best results, take with bromelain and vitamin C. Do not use with blood-thinning medications or supplements.
Taurine	1,000 to 1,500 mg once a day	Take between meals. Discontinue use if you suddenly have feelings of chest or throat tightness or if you break out in hives. Do not take with aspirin. Have your healthcare provider measure levels before starting taurine therapy.
Vitamin C	500 mg twice a day	Do not take high doses if you are prone to kidney stones or gout. High doses can also cause diarrhea.
Vitamin D$_3$	Have your blood levels measured by your healthcare provider, who will determine proper dosage.	
Vitamin E*	400 to 800 IU once a day	Take mixed tocopherols, the more active type of vitamin E. Consult your healthcare provider first if you are taking a blood thinner.
Zinc	25 mg once a day as zinc picolinate or zinc citrate	Your copper-to-zinc ratio is very important to your health. If you are taking zinc and iron supplements, take one in the morning and one in the evening. (Taking them together reduces the efficiency of both.)

*This supplement can have a blood-thinning action.

nutrients may allow you to decrease—and possibly eliminate—your dosage of diuretics while continuing to lower your blood pressure. However, you should never stop taking your blood pressure medication without your doctor's approval.

- Calcium
- Carnitine
- Coenzyme Q-10
- Fiber
- Gamma-linolenic acid (GLA)
- Hawthorn berry

- Magnesium
- Potassium
- Protein
- Taurine
- Vitamin B_6 (pyridoxine)
- Vitamin C

Direct Vasodilators

Direct vasodilators are drugs that decrease blood pressure by widening blood vessels. Yet they can cause serious side effects, including headaches, dizziness, upset stomach, and joint pain. Although these side effects may subside when the vasodilator is combined with a beta blocker medication, beta blockers can cause other problems, including worsened asthma and severe depression. Instead of taking a beta blocker with your direct vasodilator medication, try adding any of the following nutrients to your regimen. You may even find that taking the vasodilator is no longer necessary—but do not stop taking it or a beta blocker without the approval of your doctor.

- Alpha lipoic acid
- Arginine
- Calcium
- Coenzyme Q-10
- Fiber

- Garlic
- Magnesium
- Omega-3 fatty acids
- Potassium
- Soy

Angiotensin-Converting Enzyme Inhibitors

Angiotensin-converting enzyme inhibitors—or ACE Inhibitors—are vasodilators that act by restricting the production of the enzyme angiotensin II. This enzyme causes blood vessels to constrict, which results in their becoming more narrow. Restricting this enzyme allows the blood more room to move through the blood vessels, decreasing pressure. However, ACE Inhibitors can also decrease your body's store of important trace minerals such as copper, selenium, and zinc while increasing your potassium levels. The following foods and supplements can limit these side effects and increase the effectiveness of your ACE Inhibitor. You may also find it helpful to take a multivitamin.

- Casein (a phosphoprotein found in milk and cheese)
- Egg yolks
- Garlic
- Gelatin
- Hawthorn berry
- Hydrolyzed wheat germ isolate
- Hydrolyzed whey protein

- Omega-3 fatty acids
- Pycnogenol
- Sake
- Sardines
- Seaweed
- Tuna
- Zinc

Angiotensin II Receptor Blockers

Angiotensin II receptor blockers (ARBs) are vasodilators that can help lower your blood pressure by blocking the effects of the enzyme angiotensin II. ARBs are often effective for people for whom ACE inhibitors have failed. The most common side effect is dizziness, but some people also experience fever, nasal congestion, back pain, and more. The nutrients on the following list can help you avoid these possible side effects while allowing you to continue your medication. You may even find that you are able to decrease your dosage, but don't change your dosage without first consulting your healthcare provider.

- Coenzyme Q-10
- Fiber
- Gamma-linolenic acid (GLA)
- Garlic

- Potassium
- Vitamin B$_6$ (pyridoxine)
- Vitamin C

Central Alpha Agonists

By stimulating alpha-receptors in the brain, central alpha agonists widen the peripheral arteries, releasing the pressure on the blood flow. However, these medications can cause dizziness, dry mouth, sedation, and rebound hypertension, so they are usually reserved as a last resort. The following nutrients can be taken with central alpha agonists to improve their function and reduce side effects. It can also be helpful to restrict dietary sodium.

- Coenzyme Q-10
- Docosahexaenoic acid (DHA)
- Fiber
- Garlic
- Gamma-linolenic acid (GLA)
- Potassium
- Protein
- Taurine
- Zinc
- Vitamin B_6 (pyridoxine)
- Vitamin C

Calcium Channel Blockers

Calcium channel blockers decrease blood pressure by limiting the movement of calcium into the blood vessels. The negative effect of these medications is that they can change the strength of the heart muscle's contractions. The following nutrients can help counter this effect as well as lower blood pressure.

- Alpha lipoic acid
- Calcium
- Cysteine (n-acetylcysteine, or NAC)
- Garlic
- Hawthorn berry
- Magnesium
- Omega-3 fatty acids
- Vitamin B_6 (pyridoxine)
- Vitamin C
- Vitamin E

CONCLUSION

As you have seen, high blood pressure is a disease process that can cause you substantial medical problems. Both hypothyroidism and hyperthyroidism are secondary causes of hypertension. Treating thyroid disease commonly helps improve high blood pressure. Fortunately, there are numerous treatments, both medications as well as natural therapies that have clinical trials showing their efficacy in treating hypertension.

11

Thyroid Hormones and Digestive Health

As you've already learned, every biological function relies on a healthy thyroid gland, and the digestive process is no exception. Disturbances in thyroid function have numerous gastrointestinal manifestations, the true incidence of, which is unknown. Digestive symptoms or signs may also reveal clues to thyroid disease and, when ignored or underestimated, the diagnosis may be delayed, and serious consequences may occur. Additionally, individuals with thyroid dysfunction are at an increased risk of developing specific pathologies in the digestive system, whether due to thyroid hormone disturbances or associated with a particular thyroid disease.

Although many factors, from overall health to day-to-day diet, can affect digestion, normal digestion cannot take place without a well-functioning thyroid that produces appropriate amounts of thyroid hormones. Moreover, the thyroid relies on digestive health to support its own functions.

This chapter first looks at the significant connection between the thyroid and the digestive tract and examines the common problems that can occur when either system is not functioning optimally. This part of the book then explores several additional digestive problems that are related to the thyroid gland.

HOW THE THYROID AND THE DIGESTIVE TRACT INTERACT

If you've ever looked at a list of thyroid dysfunction symptoms (see Chapters 2, 3, and 4), you've likely seen several digestive problems among them. This is because by affecting the rate of metabolism—the speed with, which reactions occur within the body—the thyroid can have pronounced effects on the digestive process.

The gastrointestinal manifestations of thyroid disease are generally due to reduced motility in hypothyroidism, increased motility in hyperthyroidism, autoimmune gastritis, or esophageal compression by a thyroid process. Symptoms usually resolve with treatment of thyroid disease.

A healthy gut microbiota not only has beneficial effects on the activity of the immune system, but also on thyroid function. Thyroid and intestinal diseases prevalently coexist. Hashimoto's thyroiditis and Graves' disease are the most common autoimmune thyroid diseases and often co-exist with celiac disease and non-celiac wheat sensitivity. This is due to the damaged intestinal barrier and the subsequent increase in intestinal permeability, allowing antigens to pass more easily and activate the immune system or cross-react with extraintestinal tissues, respectively.

Dysbiosis (an imbalance between the types of organisms present in your GI tract) has not only been found in autoimmune thyroid disease, but has also been reported in thyroid carcinoma, in, which an increased number of carcinogenic and inflammatory bacterial strains were observed. Furthermore, the composition of the gut microbiota has an influence on the availability of essential micronutrients for the thyroid gland.

As you have seen, iodine, iron, and copper are crucial for thyroid hormone synthesis, selenium, and zinc are needed for converting T4 to T3, and vitamin D assists in regulating the immune response. Those micronutrients are often found to be deficient in thyroid autoimmune disease, resulting in malfunctioning of the thyroid. Moreover, bariatric surgery can lead to an inadequate absorption of these nutrients and further implicates changes in thyroid stimulating hormone (TSH) and T3 levels. Supplementation of probiotics (good bacteria) in several studies showed beneficial effects on thyroid hormones and thyroid function in general.

Hyperthyroidism

When the thyroid is overactive (hyperthyroidism), your entire body tends to run on "high." By speeding up the digestive process and peristalsis—the wave-like muscle contractions that move food through the digestive tract—hyperthyroidism tends to make the stools pass too quickly through the digestive tract. Normally, as the waste moves down the tract, a certain amount of water is removed from the waste and absorbed into the large intestines, causing the stools to become firmer, but not so firm that they can't pass easily out of the body. But transit time affects the firmness of the stools. When the waste material moves more quickly than normal, very little water has a chance to be removed, causing the stools to remain loose. This condition is referred to as diarrhea.

Digestive symptoms may represent the only manifestations of hyperthyroidism. A lack of cardinal features of the disease and the presence of persistent abdominal pain, intractable vomiting, weight loss, and altered bowel habits are designated as apathetic hyperthyroidism. Dysphagia (impairment in the production of speech) is a rare manifestation of hyperthyroidism and can have an acute or chronic pattern. It may be related to direct compression from goiter or to altered neurohormonal regulation. Excess thyroid hormone may cause myopathy (disease of the muscle tissue), which involves striated muscles of the pharynx and the upper third of the esophagus. Subsequently, the oropharyngeal (middle part of the throat behind the mouth) phase of swallowing is predominantly impaired and then the person is predisposed to nasal regurgitation and aspiration pneumonia. In the esophagus, thyroid hormone excess increases the velocity of contractions. Thyrotoxic patients may frequently complain of chronic dyspeptic symptoms such as epigastric pain (pain in upper abdomen), fullness, and belching. Hypergastrinemia—increased levels of gastrin, which aids in digestion—found in hyperthyroidism may also influence gastric and intestinal motility.

Appetite increase is common but may not be adequate to maintain weight in severe disease. Up to 25 percent of patients with hyperthyroidism have mild-to-moderate diarrhea with frequent bowel movements. In addition, some degree of fat malabsorption is usually present. A study found that patients with Graves' disease (autoimmune hyperthyroidism) were at a 5-fold added risk of developing celiac disease when compared to sex- and age-matched controls. In such cases, celiac disease may contribute to diarrhea and malabsorption. In addition, thyrotoxicosis has been reported in 3.8 percent of patients with ulcerative colitis, while the incidence of ulcerative colitis in hyperthyroid patients varies around one percent. Furthermore, thyroid disease may exacerbate ulcerative colitis symptoms or alter the response to therapy. Moreover, a positive correlation between Graves' disease and ulcerative colitis has been reported. Likewise, hyperthyroidism is accompanied by normal gastric emptying with low acid production, partly due to autoimmune gastritis with hypergastrinemia, which is increased levels of gastrin, a hormone that aids in digestion. This affects acid levels in your stomach.

Understanding the Gut

In recent years, it has become clear that a healthy digestive system is essential to overall well-being. Amazingly, the gut is home to up to 70 percent of your immune system, which is complex and beyond the scope of this book. It is significantly influenced and assisted by the 100 trillion or so bacteria, also called flora, which inhabit the gut. Without the flora, your immune system would be compromised. Unfortunately, not all gut bacteria support a strong immune system and good health. Some of the bacteria are "good," and others are "bad." Good bacteria aid in the metabolism and absorption of nutrients and help them get into the bloodstream. Bad bacteria, on the other hand, can cause painful gas, bloating, and inflammation. Worse, studies show that these less-beneficial bacteria emit chemicals that can damage the intestinal lining, leading to leaky gut syndrome, a condition in, which the lining of the small intestine becomes damaged and allows food particles, waste products, and toxins to "leak" into the bloodstream. As you'll learn, healthy gut bacteria are crucial to your well-being in another way. They assist the conversion of the thyroid hormones T4 to T3. Since T3 has about five times the hormone "strength" of T4, this substance is vital for the regulation of all metabolic processes within the body.

The 5R Program

Since gastrointestinal health, a healthy gut, is crucial for your overall health, you may want to follow this 5R program, which is sure to help you and your gut heal. Your physician can order a gut health test to make the diagnosis and can also help with the treatment. The 5R program: remove, replace, repopulate, repair, and rebalance.

Remove: Removing the source of the imbalance is the critical first step, be it pathogenic organisms or foods you are allergic to.

Replace: Replacing hydrochloric acid, digestive enzymes, bile acids, intrinsic secretions, and fiber are also very important. Acid is very important in the body. It has many functions including sterilizing the food you eat, and increasing the denaturing of proteins, which prepares the protein for breakdown by gastric and pancreatic enzymes.

Repopulate: It is important that your GI tract be repopulated with healthy bacteria. Probiotics are microbial food supplements that beneficially affect your body by improving the intestinal microbal balance. Common probiotics are *Lactobacillus*, *Bifidobacterium*, and the probiotic yeast *Saccharomyces boulardii*. Fermented food such as yogurt, tempeh, and sauerkraut are sources of microbes that may have probiotic effects. Ingesting foods that provide the fuel to feed good bacteria (prebiotics) is also important. This can be done by consuming supplements and/or intaking prebiotic foods containing a fiber called inulin. Artichoke, chicory root, leeks, garlic, and onions are all good sources.

Repair: There are nutrients that help the GI tract repair itself. Glutamine is an excellent nutrient that works on the small intestine. Glutamine stimulates the intestinal mucosal growth and protects against mucosal atrophy and plays an important role in acid-base balance in the body. Fasting has also been shown to be helpful in treating leaky gut syndrome. During fasting the white blood cell activity in the body increases, which more effectively removes circulating immune complexes from the body and decreases inflammation and leaky gut syndrome. Herbal therapies such as quercetin, which is found in onions and blue-green algae, has also been shown clinically to treat leaky gut syndrome. In addition, arginine, zinc, vitamins A, C, and D, tocopherols, carotenoids, folate, pantothenic acid, antioxidants, and omega-3 fatty acids are beneficial.

Rebalance: This is where lifestyle really comes into play. It is important to address the external stressors in your life with practices like prayer, yoga, meditation, deep breathing, good sleep, and other mindfulness-based practices.

Hypothyroidism

On the other hand, when the thyroid is underactive (hypothyroidism), all the processes in the body, including the digestive process, tend to slow down. When waste moves through the digestive tract too slowly, with the body absorbing more and more water along the way, the stools become hard and dry, and passing them becomes difficult and painful. This condition is referred to as constipation.

A Healthy Gut

You've now seen how an overactive or underactive thyroid can affect the bowel. But the bowel (or gut) can also influence the function of the thyroid gland. You may remember from Chapter 1 that the thyroid produces more of the T4 hormone than the T3. It then relies on other organs and body systems to convert T4 into T3. About 20 percent of this conversion takes place in the gut. Scientists don't know the precise chain of events that allow this vital conversion to take place, but they have found that healthy gut flora ("good" bacteria) aid the conversions of T4 to T3. (To learn more about gut bacteria, see the inset on page 238.) Bad bacteria, however, may result in thyroid levels that are not as high as they should be. So, the thyroid needs the gut just as the gut needs the thyroid.

The interaction between the gut and the thyroid is complex. For instance, the gut must be healthy enough to absorb the nutrients needed by the thyroid to do its job. If the digestive system is experiencing inflammation and can't absorb the nutrients iodine and selenium, both of, which are crucial to thyroid function, the production of T3 and T4 will be reduced, and the metabolism—including digestive function—will slow.

If you are experiencing digestive problems that are not responding to treatment, it makes sense to get your thyroid function checked. Resolving any thyroid issues can be an essential part of restoring normal digestive function. Similarly, in the medical literature is now something called the thyroid-gut-axis, which discusses the importance of the influence that the gut microbiota has on thyroid function.

The results of a recent animal study reveal that there were significant differences in alpha and beta diversities of gut microbiota between primary hypothyroidism patients and healthy individuals. Four intestinal bacteria (*Veillonella, Paraprevotella, Neisseria, and Rheinheimera*) were shown to be able to distinguish untreated primary hypothyroidism patients from healthy individuals with accuracy. In addition, the short chain fatty acid producing ability of the primary hypothyroidism patients' gut was significantly decreased, which resulted in increased serum lipopolysaccharide (LPS) levels. The trial also showed that mice receiving a fecal transplant from primary hypothyroidism patients displayed decreased total thyroxine levels and suggested that primary hypothyroidism causes changes in gut microbiome. Conversely, an altered flora can affect thyroid function. In addition, bariatric surgery can lead to an inadequate absorption of important nutrients, which further causes changes in thyroid stimulating hormone (TSH) and T3 levels.

Therefore, you'll want to make sure to safeguard your digestive health so that your thyroid is able to get the support it needs.

ACID REFLUX DISEASE

Patients with hypothyroidism (an insufficient production of thyroid hormones) often take antacids because they experience acid reflux, a condition in, which the acidic gastric fluid flows up from the stomach into the esophagus, causing a burning chest pain called heartburn. If these symptoms occur more than twice a week, the disorder is called acid reflux disease or gastroesophageal reflex disease (GERD).

Studies have shown that 40 percent of individuals with acid reflux have the disease because they have too little stomach acid instead of too much. In addition, Hashimoto's disease, the most common cause of hypothyroidism, may be associated with an esophageal motility disorder presenting as dysphagia or heartburn. Dyspepsia (indigestion), nausea, or vomiting may be due to delayed gastric emptying. Abdominal discomfort, flatulence, and bloating occur in those with bacterial overgrowth and improve with probiotics. Sometimes antibiotic therapy along with probiotics are needed. Reduced acid production may be due to autoimmune gastritis or low gastrin levels.

How Hypothyroidism Affects the Esophagus

To understand what is happening, you must know a little about digestive physiology. A long muscular tube called the esophagus connects the stomach to the throat. Normally, a ring-shaped sphincter muscle called the lower esophageal sphincter (LES)—found at the lowest part of the esophagus, where the tube meets the stomach—prevents the acids in the stomach, as well as other stomach contents, from moving up the esophagus into the throat. (See Figure 11.1 on page 242.) But when someone is hypothyroid, both this sphincter and the one at the top of the esophagus (known as the upper esophageal sphincter, or UES) become lax and don't close properly. This enables the stomach contents—including stomach acids—to flow upwards into the esophagus. Because hypothyroidism slows the speed at, which all activities in the body take place (decrease esophageal peristalsis), it has been shown to delay gastric emptying, which means that there is more acid present to flow into the esophagus. In addition to heartburn, symptoms of acid reflux can include chest pain, difficulty breathing, difficulty swallowing, hoarseness, sore throat, a dry cough, and the regurgitation of food or a sour liquid. When the proximal portion of the esophagus is involved, myxedema (a severe form of hypothyroidism characterized by swelling and thickening of the skin) causes oropharyngeal dysphagia (difficulty or discomfort in swallowing), while esophagitis and hiatal hernia occur when the distal (last part) esophagus is altered. Esophageal motility disorders reduced velocity and amplitude of esophageal peristalsis and a decrease in lower sphincter pressure all contribute to dysphagia (difficulty or discomfort in swallowing). Additionally, gastric dysmotility is significantly more frequent in hypothyroid patients and is a result of muscle edema (swelling) and altered myoelectrical activity. The hypothyroid state seems to delay gastric emptying. Achlorhydria (lack of stomach acid) in hypothyroidism may be related to subnormal serum gastrin.

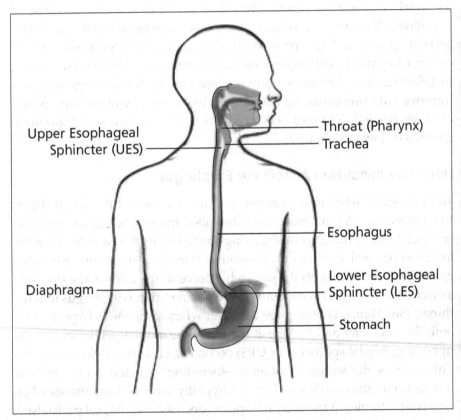

Figure 11.1. The Esophagus

Treatment

Believing that the stomach is producing too much stomach acid, hypothyroid patients often take antacids. Unfortunately, this approach does not always help, as the problem isn't always an overproduction of acid. In fact, hypothyroid patients are often found to be abnormally low in the hormone gastrin, which stimulates the secretion of gastric acid, and to also have lower levels of stomach acid than healthy people. By further lowering the acid in the stomach, antacids and other medications can create an environment in, which food is not properly broken down and absorbed, and nutrient deficiencies—including deficiencies of the nutrients needed to produce thyroid hormones—result. Moreover, levothyroxine, a medication used to treat hypothyroidism, requires stomach acid to become a bioidentical form of the thyroid hormone T4. If you have low stomach acid, either because of hypothyroidism or because of antacids, you may find that this medication may not be as beneficial as it could be.

HELICOBACTER PYLORI [H. PYLORI]

For some people with hypothyroidism, heartburn may be caused or exacerbated by an infection of *Helicobacter pylori,* or *H. pylori,* the most common chronic bacterial pathogen found in human beings. Researchers are not sure of the mechanism that causes so many people with hypothyroidism to have *H. pylori* infections.

Helicobacter pylori and Hypothyroidism

Some studies have indicated that this bacterium may trigger autoimmune disorders such as Hashimoto's thyroiditis, the most common cause of hypothyroidism in the United States. Certainly, more people with Hashimoto's disease are affected by *H. pylori* than people in the general population. It is also known that acid-reducing medications, which are often taken by people with hypothyroidism, create an ideal condition for *H. pylori* to thrive. One five-year study published in *The New England Journal of Medicine* found that rates of *H. pylori* increased from 59 percent to 81 percent in patients taking one over-the-counter acid-reducing medication. Heartburn is just one possible symptom associated with these bacteria. Other symptoms, ranging from bloating to burning abdominal pain, may also be present. (See the inset on page 244 to learn more about *Helicobacter pylori* bacteria.)

Helicobacter Pylori—
An Underdiagnosed Digestive Villain

On page 243, you learned that *Helicobacter pylori*—a bacteria that can cause infection of the stomach—can result in heartburn and other digestive problems. You also learned that this is one of the most common infections worldwide, and that it is more common in people with thyroid dysfunction than it is in the general population. But despite its prevalence, it too often goes undiagnosed.

Part of the explanation for the under-recognition of *H. pylori* is the fact that in some people, it causes no symptoms. In these cases, the infection, which usually occurs because of food-borne bacteria or contaminated utensils, remains localized in the gastric area at so low a level that no one is aware of its presence. In other people, though, the bacteria can lead to several distressing problems, including abdominal pain, acid reflux, bloating, nausea, vomiting, loss of appetite, and loss of weight. Sometimes, these symptoms indicate serious disorders. *H. pylori* is, in fact, present in 60 to 100 percent of patients with gastric ulcers, and 90 to 100 percent of patients with duodenal ulcers. Moreover, it is associated with stomach cancer and lymphoma. Furthermore, *H. pylori* infection has been proposed to imitate the antigenic components of the thyroid cell membrane and may play a leading role in the onset of autoimmune diseases, such as Hashimoto's thyroiditis.

Because infection with *H. pylori* is so common, in the absence of symptoms, doctors often recommend no treatment whatsoever. But since this organism sometimes results in serious conditions, physicians are becoming increasingly interested in diagnosing and treating it. Several diagnostic tests are now available: endoscopy, a breath test, a blood test, and a very accurate fecal antigen test. Once diagnosed, an *H. pylori* infection is generally treated with a combination of antibiotics and a proton pump inhibitor. In some cases, the combination of zinc and the amino acid carnosine are also used to treat *H. pylori* as are other nutrients.

If you are experiencing any of the symptoms of *H. pylori,* be sure to get tested for this common bacterium. If the test is positive, remember that this bacterium can have nasty consequences, so it pays to get prompt treatment.

Treatment

The good news is that the acid reflux associated with hypothyroidism can often be relieved. When thyroid hormone is used to treat hypothyroidism and levels of T3 and T4 are returned to normal, appropriate tension of the lower esophageal sphincter is commonly restored. This prevents stomach acid from escaping into the esophagus. Treatment with thyroid hormone also causes the levels of gastrin and stomach acid to normalize. When *H. pylori* is the problem, antibiotics usually offer a solution, and heartburn disappears along with the infection. There are also nutritional therapies you can take in addition to antibiotics to help resolve the *H. pylori* such as zinc carnosine. Remember when taking an antibiotic, you must also take a probiotic. However, do not take them at the same time. Take the antibiotic and then wait at least two hours to take the probiotic.

If you are suffering from chronic acid reflux, keep in mind that this disorder is not always caused by the overproduction of stomach acids, and that antacids and similar medications may not be the answer. If you have been diagnosed with thyroid disease, you may find that correcting your thyroid dysfunction also soothes your digestive tract. People with thyroid disorders are seldom tested for *H. pylori* even when symptoms are present, so be sure that your physician considers all possible causes and their treatments.

Intestine and Colon

In hypothyroidism, appetite is usually reduced, but weight gain may reach 10 percent because of fluid retention. Vague abdominal discomfort and bloating may be erroneously attributed to functional bowel disease. The effect of hypothyroidism on the gastrointestinal tract appears to be multifactorial with possible alterations in hormone receptors, neuromuscular disorders, and myopathy caused by infiltration of the intestinal wall. Reduction of peristalsis in hypothyroidism is the main pathophysiologic process and constipation remains the most frequent gastrointestinal complaint. Up to 15 percent of people have less than three bowel movements a week; whereas perfect bowel function is two bowel movements a day. Moreover, thyroid hormone deficiency may influence transepithelial flux transport by inhibiting anion exchange (a chemical process in, which anions—negatively charged ions—are exchanged or removed) with a subsequent effect on intestinal motility.

Furthermore, hypothyroidism may be associated with a decrease in duodenal basal electrical rhythm, which allows the smooth muscle cell to depolarize and contract rhythmically when exposed to hormonal signals. Although rare, severe cases of hypothyroidism can lead to an ileus or rarely a pseudo-obstruction with fecal impaction and megacolon (an abnormal dilation of the colon). Inadvertent surgery in these situations is harmful and may be lethal. Absorption of specific substances may be decreased, but the total quantity absorbed is usually normal or increased due to an extended time in bowel transit. Diarrhea in the hypothyroid state is mainly the result of increased bacterial growth secondary to bowel hypomotility—decreased peristalsis.

CELIAC DISEASE

Another way in, which thyroid disease is connected to digestive health is through the incidence of celiac disease. Celiac disease is an autoimmune disorder that manifests itself when people eat gluten, a protein found in wheat, barley, rye, and products made from these ingredients. When the gluten reaches the digestive tract, an immune response is triggered in the small intestine, causing symptoms that can include diarrhea, bloating, fatigue, abdominal pain, and weight loss. Over time, this causes inflammation of the lining of the small intestine and prevents nutrients from being adequately absorbed, a condition known as malabsorption.

Celiac Disease and Thyroid Disease

A significant number of people with celiac disease have autoimmune thyroid disease (ATD)—either Hashimoto's disease (a frequent type of hypothyroidism) or Graves' disease (the most common form of hyperthyroidism). In fact, people with celiac disease are nearly four times more likely to develop an autoimmune thyroid condition than people who do not have celiac disease. The reverse also holds true: people with autoimmune thyroid disease are far more likely to develop celiac disease than the general public. In one study conducted by Dr. Alessio Fasano, a celiac disease researcher, half of the people newly diagnosed with celiac disease also had a dysfunctional thyroid.

So far, scientists aren't sure why the connection exists between autoimmune thyroid disease and celiac. Some have hypothesized that people with celiac disease and autoimmune thyroid disorders share a genetic predisposition. Some have observed that the anti-tTG antibodies that are present in people with active celiac disease also bind and react to thyroid tissue and may stimulate the development of autoimmune thyroid

Following a Gluten-Free Diet

As you learned on page 243, people who have an autoimmune thyroid disorder can often benefit from following a gluten-free diet. And, of course, anyone with celiac disease or gluten sensitivity *must* stick to gluten-free foods. The following gluten-containing grains and grain-based products need to be avoided on a gluten-free diet:

- Barley
- Bulgur wheat
- Couscous (usually made from wheat)
- Einkorn (a type of wheat)
- Kamut (a type of wheat)
- Pasta made from wheat, rye, or barley.

- Rye
- Semolina (the hard part of wheat)
- Spelt (a type of wheat)
- Triticale (a wheat hybrid)
- Wheat

The following grains and grain substitutes may be consumed on a gluten-free diet:

- Almond flour
- Amaranth
- Buckwheat
- Coconut flour
- Corn
- Cornstarch

- Millet
- Potato flour
- Quinoa
- Rice (white, brown, and wild)
- Sorghum
- Teff

In addition to avoiding gluten-containing grains and flours, it is essential to become aware of processed products that contain ingredients made from these grains. Most soy sauce, for instance, is made with fermented wheat, so you'll need to look for a gluten-free brand. Many sauces and soups and some condiments, even some types of ketchup and mustard, contain gluten-based thickeners. Since naturally gluten-free, oats often become cross-contaminated during processing, you'll need to search out brands that are made for people who can't have gluten. Read food package labels carefully for statements about gluten, and if in doubt, contact the manufacturer for more information.

disease. Healthcare providers that specialize in Anti-Aging and Personalized Medicine believe people who develop Hashimoto's thyroid disease are triggered by underlying celiac disease or gluten sensitivity. Whatever the mechanism involved—the connection between autoimmune thyroid disease and celiac disease has been well established by study after study.

Treatment

Fortunately, just as thyroid autoimmune disease and celiac disease are interrelated, a similar method of management appears to offer relief to people with both disorders. A gluten-free diet is essential to people with celiac disease and gluten sensitivity. When people with celiac follow this diet, their anti-tTG antibodies—which indicate that the disease is present and active—decrease and may eventually disappear. When people with autoimmune thyroid disease follow a gluten-free diet, their thyroid antibody levels commonly decline. In some cases, when people with both celiac and Hashimoto's have followed a gluten-free diet, thyroid function has returned to normal, and the individuals have no longer needed thyroid medication. Although this type of complete recovery is rare—usually, autoimmune diseases require lifelong treatment—many clinicians have stated that a gluten-free diet is essential for those with autoimmune thyroid disease.

If you have an autoimmune thyroid disorder—Hashimoto's or Graves'—it is important to be tested for celiac disease. People with celiac do not always experience digestive upset, especially at the onset on the disease, so even if you feel that your digestion is working well, a test for celiac may be able to provide more information about your condition. Considering the evidence, it also makes sense to try a gluten-free diet. (See the inset on page 247.) For most people with autoimmune thyroid disease, excluding gluten has proven essential to help optimize their thyroid function.

Another influencing factor of the microbiota is its effect on neurotransmitters such as dopamine, which can inhibit thyroid stimulating hormone (TSH). In fact, recent research has demonstrated that neurotransmitters can play a significant role in gastrointestinal (GI) physiology. Norepinephrine (NE), epinephrine (E), dopamine, and serotonin have recently been topics of interest because of their roles in gut physiology and their potential roles in gastrointestinal and central nervous system pathophysiology. These neurotransmitters are able to regulate and control not only blood flow, but also affect gut motility, nutrient absorption, gastrointestinal innate immune system, and the microbiome.

Autoimmune Thyroid Studies and the GI Tract

A healthy gut microbiota not only has beneficial effects on the activity of the immune system but also on thyroid function particularly in thyroid autoimmune diseases, such as Hashimoto's thyroiditis and Graves' disease. This can be explained by the damaged intestinal barrier and the subsequent increase in intestinal permeability, allowing antigens to pass more easily and activate the immune system or cross-react with extraintestinal tissues, respectively. Dysbiosis has not only been found in thyroid autoimmune disease but has also been reported in thyroid cancer, in, which an increased number of carcinogenic and inflammatory bacterial strains are seen. In other words, the negative influence on the immune system and the inflammatory regulation of an impaired microbiota appears to promote autoimmune diseases, such as autoimmune thyroid disorders as well as cancer.

Likewise, the interaction between genetic susceptibility, epigenetic (changes in organisms caused by modification of gene expression rather than alteration of the genetic code itself), endogenous, and environmental factors play a key role in the initiation and progression of autoimmune thyroid diseases. Consequently, studies have shown that gut microbiota alterations take part in the development of autoimmune diseases. Furthermore, beta diversity analysis (measures distance or dissimilarity between each sample pair) showed that gut microbiota from autoimmune thyroid patients was different than healthy controls. A study demonstrated that gut dysbiosis in autoimmune thyroid disease patients may contribute to thyroid disease development. Thus, gut dysbiosis (imbalance of microorganisms in the intestines) may be related to a dysfunctional immune system response in autoimmune thyroid disease patients. It also may be related to the loss of tolerance to self-antigens including thyroglobulin and the autoimmunity that triggers Hashimoto's thyroiditis and Graves' disease. Another study revealed that an altered microbiota composition increases the prevalence of Hashimoto's. There was a decline in abundance of *Prevotella9* and *Dialister* bacteria, while elevated genera of the diseased group included *Escherichia-Shigella* and *Parasutterella* bacteria. The alteration in gut microbial configuration was also monitored at the species level, which showed an increased abundance of *E. coli* in Hashimoto's thyroiditis.

Furthermore, microbes influence thyroid hormone levels by regulating iodine uptake, degradation, and enterohepatic cycling, which is a feedback mechanism resulting from the combined roles of the liver and the intestine. In addition, there is a pronounced influence of minerals on interactions between the host and microbiota, particularly selenium, iron, and zinc. Moreover, in manifested thyroid disorders, the microbiota may affect L-thyroxine uptake and influence the action of propylthiouracil—used to treat Graves' disease. Furthermore, the relative analysis of richness indices and diversity illustrated lesser diversification of intestinal bacteria in Graves' disease patients in contrast to controls in the same study. The data statistics showed the alteration in phyla of Graves' disease as compared to controls. At the family taxonomic level, the relative abundance of *Prevotellaceae* and *Pasteurellaceae* were significantly higher in patients, while *Enterobacteriaceae, Veillonellaceae,* and *Rikenellaceae* were significantly lower in the diseased group as compared to the control. At the genus level, a significant raise in genera count of the diseased group were *Prevotella9* and *Haemophilus*, while significantly decreased in the genera of the Graves' group were *Alistipes* and *Faecalibacterium*. The modulation in intestinal bacterial composition was also observed at the species level, particularly *H. parainfluenza* abundance was raised in Graves' disease. The outcomes of the study agreed with the hypothesis of gut microbial dysbiosis in Graves' disease.

Thus, the consequences of these two thyroid autoimmune diseases affect the entire metabolism of the human body.

Treatment

As you have seen in the chapters on Hashimoto's thyroiditis and Graves' disease there are several therapies that may be needed depending on the severity of the disease process. It is imperative that no matter what treatments are chosen for these autoimmune diseases, the GI tract health be normalized in order to have the best therapeutic outcome.

CONCLUSION

If you have been diagnosed with hypothyroidism or hyperthyroidism, it is paramount that you get the treatment you need. This alone may relieve your digestive problems. If you have not been diagnosed with thyroid dysfunction but are experiencing one or more digestive issues, be aware that thyroid disorders are a common cause and should be considered. Also recognize that a range of other issues, such as infection by *H. pylori* bacteria, can cause GI problems. By understanding the potential culprits, you'll be better prepared to search for the cause of your digestive disorder. Sometimes, it is necessary to use a combination of treatments to experience optimal digestive health. For instance, to resolve issues such as diarrhea or constipation, you may need to pair treatment for thyroid dysfunction with a healthier diet. Supplementation with probiotics has also been shown to have beneficial effects on thyroid hormone levels and thyroid function. By using a treatment program developed by a qualified healthcare provider in Personalized/Anti-Aging Medicine who is aware of all your medical issues, you can enhance thyroid function, improve your digestion, and safeguard your overall health.

12

Hypothyroidism and Nonalcoholic Fatty Liver Disease

onalcoholic fatty liver disease (NAFLD) is one of the most frequent chronic hepatic (liver) conditions worldwide. NAFLD occurs in approximately 10 to 30 percent of people in the world and in 58 percent to 74 percent of people that are obese. Moreover, between 75 million and 100 million individuals in the United States are estimated to have nonalcoholic fatty liver disease. Furthermore, 66 percent of patients older than 50 years with diabetes or obesity are thought to have nonalcoholic steatohepatitis (a liver condition caused by liver swelling, which is an advanced stage of fatty liver disease) with advanced fibrosis. The spectrum of nonalcoholic fatty liver disease goes from hepatic steatosis (deposition of fat in the liver) to steatohepatitis, cirrhosis, and hepatocellular carcinoma (liver cancer). The incidence of nonalcoholic fatty liver disease-related hepatocellular carcinoma is increasing and up to 50 percent of cases may occur in the absence of cirrhosis. In patients with nonalcoholic steatohepatitis, half of deaths are due to cardiovascular disease and malignancy, yet the general public has not been made aware of this. Moreover, cirrhosis, the third leading cause of death in patients with nonalcoholic fatty liver disease, is predicted to become the most common indication for liver transplantation in the near future.

There are two forms of NAFLD:

1. Nonalcoholic fatty liver (NAFL), defined as 5 percent or greater hepatic steatosis without hepatocellular injury or fibrosis

2. Nonalcoholic steatohepatitis (NASH), defined as 5 percent or greater

hepatic steatosis plus hepatocellular injury and inflammation, with or without fibrosis.

NASH can progress to cirrhosis, fibrosis, or hepatocellular carcinoma. If no inflammation is present in patients with hepatic steatosis, then usually there is not progression to a more severe hepatic disease. However, if the individual has NAFLD, they do have an increased risk of developing cardiovascular disease and there is also an elevated risk of all-cause mortality. Furthermore, if the person has hepatic steatosis this may increase the risk of progression to other diseases of the liver such as hepatitis C.

RISK FACTORS

The following risk factors for the development of nonalcoholic fatty liver disease include:

- Hypertriglyceridemia (high triglycerides)
- Metabolic syndrome (It is a cluster of conditions that occur together, increasing your risk of heart disease, stroke, and type 2 diabetes. These conditions include increased blood pressure, high blood sugar, excess body fat around the waist, and abnormal cholesterol and/or triglyceride levels.)
- Obesity
- Type 2 diabetes

CAUSES

The pathogenesis of NAFLD is related to several things:

- NAFLD is characterized by excess accumulation of triglyceride in the hepatocyte due to both increased inflow of free fatty acids and hepatic lipogenesis (biochemical process of synthesizing fatty acids).
- Insulin resistance is the major mechanism in the development and progression of NAFLD/nonalcoholic steatohepatitis (NASH).
- There is strong evidence that mitochondrial dysfunction plays a significant role in the development and progression of nonalcoholic fatty liver disease. Impaired mitochondrial fatty acid oxidation and a reduction

in mitochondrial quality have been suggested to play a major role In NAFLD development and progression. In fact, mitochondria make up to 18 percent of the total volume of hepatocytes and play a critical role in the liver's metabolic functions as well as nutrient (carbohydrates, lipids, and proteins) oxidation for energy generation.

- Metabolic oxidative stress, autophagy (process where cells break down and destroys old, damaged, or abnormal proteins and other substances in its cytoplasm), and inflammation induce NASH progression. In addition, an increase in ROS (reactive oxygen species) production that occurs in oxidative stress leads to hepatocyte damage and inflammation. Since patients with hypothyroidism have elevated markers of oxidative stress, oxidative stress in these individuals could be the cause of cellular damage in liver tissue by reducing β-oxidation of fatty acids and increasing peroxidation of lipids. This is the process in, which free radicals "steal" electrons from the lipids in cell membranes, resulting in cell damage. Furthermore, TSH stimulates hepatic gluconeogenesis (formation of glucose) and causes hypercholesterolemia (high cholesterol), ultimately leading to the development and progression of NAFLD.

- Also, some authors have suggested that high sugar intake increases the risk of developing NAFLD.

- Furthermore, high fructose corn syrup is also proposed by some researchers as a causative factor for nonalcoholic fatty liver disease.

- Hypothyroidism-induced or hypothyroidism-associated NAFLD is receiving more attention. This form of NAFLD has generally been attributed to reduced thyroid hormone signaling in the liver, resulting in decreased hepatic lipid utilization and secondary lipid accumulation. In a recent study, people with low thyroid function were significantly more likely to have NADH and approximately twice as likely to have advanced liver fibrosis than those with optimal thyroid function.

- Furthermore, risks of developing NASH and advanced fibrosis increased significantly with high plasma concentration of TSH. Likewise, thyroid hormones are totally involved in the regulation of body weight, lipid metabolism, and insulin resistance. Therefore, thyroid hormones play a role in the pathogenesis of nonalcoholic fatty liver disease and nonalcoholic steatohepatitis (NASH). In fact, thyroid dysfunctions in the form of overt or subclinical hypothyroidism are prevalent among individuals with NAFLD/NASH in clinical trials.

- One study examined twenty-six studies involving over 61,000 people. NAFLD/NASH patients had significantly higher TSH levels than controls in adults. Consequently, although the main reason for NASH in individuals with hypothyroidism is a decrease in thyroid hormone levels, elevated TSH, regardless of thyroid hormone levels, could also affect the development of NAFLD.

TREATMENT

Conventional treatments include ursodeoxycholic acid, which is a naturally occurring bile acid, and weight loss if the patient is obese. Exercise is also important. Other treatments, such as bariatric surgery (least optimal treatment since it causes nutritional depletions), vitamin E supplements, and pharmacologic therapy with thiazolidinediones or glucagon-like peptide-1 analogues, have shown potential benefit. However, the data are limited and therefore these therapies are not considered routine treatments. In addition, the primary and secondary prevention of NAFLD may require aggressive strategies for managing obesity, diabetes, and metabolic syndrome.

Personalized Medicine Therapies

A Personalized Medicine approach is centered around dietary factors and nutritional supplements.

Diet

- Lifestyle modification is the cornerstone of treatment of all patients with NAFLD, regardless of disease stage. Most people with NAFLD benefit from weight loss.

- Studies have shown a decrease in hepatic steatosis and fibrosis with weight loss in patients that were overweight. Among those who achieved a greater than or equal to 1percent total body weight reduction, 9 percent experienced resolution of NASH, 100 percent had a reduction in NAFLD activity score, and 45 percent had regression of fibrosis.

- It is important to discontinue intake of high fructose corn syrup. Fructose is rapidly taken up by hepatocytes after ingestion and unlike glucose its conversion to fructose-1-phosphase is not rate limited. This leads to ATP—adenosine triphosphate production—depletion, ATP enhanced endoplasmic reticulum stress—ER stress (when the capacity of the ER to fold proteins becomes saturated), mitochondrial dysfunction, and potentially hepatic inflammation and injury.

- Decrease sugar intake.

- A Mediterranean diet has been shown to reduce hepatic steatosis in patients with nonalcoholic fatty liver disease. Therefore, eat a Mediterranean diet.

- If you have celiac disease, avoiding gluten has been shown to decrease fatty liver.

- Avoiding trans-fatty acids may decrease the risk of developing NAFLD.

- Brominated vegetable oil that is present in Mountain Dew and some Gatorade flavors may increase fatty liver infiltration. Consequently, avoid brominated vegetable oil.

- Intake of whey protein has been shown to improve liver function and decrease hepatic steatosis.

Exercise

- Aerobic training exercise, even in the absence of weight loss, can improve NAFLD. Moreover, aerobic exercise decreases aminotransferase levels in individuals with NAFLD.

- Further, several studies have demonstrated the benefit of aerobic exercise on radiographic NAFLD. Both 30-to-45-minute cycling sessions, or 9minutes of brisk walking or jogging three times a week improved hepatic triglyceride content.

Nutritional Supplements

- Alpha lipoic acid

  o Chronic alpha lipoic acid supplementation prevented NAFLD through multiple mechanisms by reducing steatosis, oxidative stress, immune activation, and inflammation in the liver in an animal study.

  o This is a great nutrient for mitochondrial support.

- o Dose: 200 to 300 mg daily.

- Betaine
  - o Betaine is a metabolite of choline and is a methyl donor.

  - o A study showed that 20 grams a day of betaine improved histological and biochemical parameters in individuals with NASH.

  - o Wheat germ, beets, spinach, and bran are high in betaine, or you can take a supplement.

  - o Do not take it if you have an active peptic ulcer.

- Biotin
  - o Biotin supplementation may be helpful. Biotin is made in your GI tract. If your gut is not healthy, then your body is commonly low in this important B vitamin.

- Choline
  - o Choline is a methyl donor. If an individual does not have enough methyl groups, then the body does not metabolize fat well in the liver.

  - o If a person has a genetic polymorphism (phosphatidylethanolamine N-methyltransferase) that is common, which involves an enzyme used in the biosynthesis of choline, it predisposes them to NAFLD or damage to their muscles if they do not have enough choline in their diet. About 75 percent of people are heterozygous (having two different forms of a gene) or homozygous (two identical forms of a gene) for the 744G-C polymorphism. The development of NAFLD in patients with this polymorphism has only been seen in women.

  - o Dose: 250 to 1,000 mg daily.

  - o Do not supplement with choline if you have an elevated TMAO level. Therefore, have your healthcare provider measure TMAO (a blood study) before taking choline. If you have an elevated TMAO level, and you take choline, it will increase your risk of developing heart disease.

- Coenzyme Q-10
  - o A study suggested that CoQ-10 supplemented at a dosage of 100 mg a day could be effective for improving the systemic inflammation and

biochemical variables in NAFLD. It resulted in a significant decrease in liver aminotransferases (aspartate aminotransferase [AST] and gamma-glutamyl transpeptidase [GGT]), high-sensitivity C-reactive protein (hs-CRP), tumor necrosis factor alpha (TNF-alpha), and the grades of NAFLD in the CoQ-10 group in comparison to the control group. In addition, patients who received the CoQ-10 supplement had higher serum levels of adiponectin (a hormone your fat tissue releases that helps with insulin sensitivity and inflammation) and considerable changes in serum leptin, which is a hormone your adipose tissue releases that helps your body maintain your normal weight on a long-term basis.

○ Coenzyme Q-10 supports mitochondria.

○ Dose: 300 to 400 mg a day.

• Copper

○ Animals fed a high fructose diet were shown to be low in copper.

○ Consider supplementing with a small dose of copper, particularly if you are also taking zinc. Not all people can take copper. Contact your healthcare provider if you are considering taking more copper than is commonly found in a multivitamin.

• Elevated iron levels

○ Elevated ferritin (iron) levels may be seen in about 25 percent of patients with nonalcoholic fatty liver disease. Have your healthcare provider measure your ferritin levels. If elevated, your doctor or other healthcare provider will have you donate blood on a regular basis. Do not take supplemental iron unless instructed by your doctor.

• Glutathione

○ Twenty-nine patients completed a study. Liver enzyme levels significantly decreased following treatment with glutathione for 4 months. In addition, triglycerides, non-esterified fatty acids, and ferritin levels also decreased with glutathione treatment. This pilot study demonstrated the potential therapeutic effects of oral administration of glutathione in a practical dose for patients with NAFLD.

○ Oral administration of glutathione must be in the liposomal form. Dose: one teaspoon a day or one 300 mg capsule. Glutathione can also be given IV to you by your doctor.

- Inflammation

  o Excess free fatty acids and chronic low-grade inflammation from visceral adipose tissue (VAT) are two of the most important factors contributing to liver injury progression in NAFLD. In addition, secretion of adipokines (cytokines secreted by adipose tissue that may contribute to inflammation related to obesity) from VAT, as well as lipid accumulation in the liver, further promotes inflammation through nuclear factor kappa B signaling pathways, which are also activated by free fatty acids, and contribute to insulin resistance.

  o Discuss with your doctor the use of prescription compounded low-dose naltrexone (LDN) to decrease inflammation. (See page 70.)

- Inositol

  o Studies have revealed that giving inositol has prevented experimentally induced fatty liver in both humans and animals.

  o Eat foods that have a high inositol content, such as nuts, beans, and fruits, and supplement if needed.

- L-Carnitine

  o Carnitine is responsible for transport of fatty acids into the mitochondria, which plays a role in fat metabolism.

  o It is a nutrient that benefits the mitochondria.

  o A study showed that supplementing with 1 gram, twice a day, of carnitine was beneficial.

  o Have your doctor or other healthcare provider measure TMAO levels before supplementing with carnitine.

- Lysine

  o Eating a low lysine diet may increase the risk of developing NAFLD.

  o Have your doctor measure lysine levels and increase your intake of lysine rich foods and/or supplement with lysine if your levels are low. If lysine is supplemented long-term, then take with arginine.

- Magnesium

  o A trial suggested that high intake of magnesium may be associated with reduced risks of fatty liver disease and prediabetes.

○ In addition, since the patients with NAFLD experiences oxidative stress and mitochondrial damage, supplementing with magnesium may be beneficial.

○ Also, individuals with NAFLD may be low in magnesium. Have your doctor measure RBC magnesium levels. If your levels are low, your healthcare provider will suggest the dose that is right for you. A common dose of magnesium is 400 mg a day of magnesium glycinate or magnesium threonate.

- Manganese
  ○ Supplementing with manganese, if levels are low, may be helpful.

- Omega-3 fatty acids
  ○ Several studies have shown that supplementing with omega-3 fatty acids has been beneficial in patients with NAFLD. Dose: 3,000 mg a day.

- Probiotics
  ○ Small bowel overgrowth may contribute to NAFLD.

  ○ Studies have shown that taking probiotics has been helpful to decrease hepatic steatosis.

  ○ Pantothenic acid and pantethine (vitamin B5)

  ○ Pantethine is a metabolite of pantothenic acid and plays a role in the metabolism of fat.

  ○ An uncontrolled trial showed that 600 mg of pantethine for 6 months resolved fatty liver in 9 of 16 patients studied. This is a very high dose of pantothenic acid. Only take it under a doctor's direction.

- Taurine
  ○ Taurine is an amino acid. Taurine supplementation may be beneficial since it helps to reverse hepatic steatosis by promoting the secretion of triglycerides from the liver.

  ○ Taurine has also been shown to help treat nonalcoholic fatty liver disease by decreasing the severity of oxidative stress-induced liver injury.

  ○ Have your doctor measure taurine levels and supplement according to lab levels.

o A common reason to have low taurine is long-term stress.

- Thyroid hormone replacement

  o Thyroid hormone replacement has been shown to be beneficial in people with suboptimal thyroid levels. Hypothyroidism-induced or hypothyroidism-associated NAFD is receiving more attention in the medical literature.

  o Also, thyroid hormones modify lipid accumulation in the liver, affecting leptin and adiponectin; cytokines that also have significance in the pathogenesis of hepatic steatosis. Leptin stimulates beta-oxidation and suppresses lipogenesis, while an inverse correlation (negative relationship) has been found in many studies to exist between adiponectin, triglyceride, and LDL (bad) cholesterol.

  o In addition, hypothyroidism is associated with impaired glucose and insulin metabolism, which as previously discussed, is a major risk factor for NAFLD. Also, insulin resistance leads to decreased responsiveness of glucose uptake in muscle and fat tissues, and to insulin further negatively impacting your lipid profile.

  o Consequently, have your primary care doctor, endocrinologist, or other healthcare provider measure your thyroid studies and consider thyroid hormone replacement therapy to optimize your blood levels.

- Tocotrienols

  o Tocotrienols are a special kind of vitamin E. Supplementation has been shown to decrease fatty liver.

- Vitamin B_6

  o Supplementing with B complex, including vitamin B_6, may be beneficial in people with nonalcoholic fatty liver disease. B vitamins are water soluble and leave the body quickly. Therefore, divide the dose and take one-half in the morning and one-half in the evening.

- Vitamin B_{12}

  o A study on rats showed that giving B_{12} reduced the degree of fatty infiltration and fibrosis of the liver. Therefore, consider supplementing with vitamin B_{12} and B complex twice a day in divided doses.

- Vitamins C and E

  - Studies have shown that vitamin E with or without vitamin C improved liver function studies and decreased steatosis of the liver, fibrosis, and inflammation.

- Zinc

  - Lab animals fed a low zinc diet developed fatty liver disease. Therefore, consider supplementing with zinc 15 to 5mg a day. When supplementing with zinc, also supplement with copper: 1to 15 mg of zinc to one mg of copper.

New Treatments in Trial Phase

Special attention should be given to people with NAFLD and hypothyroidism, specifically in obese or overweight individuals. Both diseases should be taken into consideration when choosing the right therapeutic modality. Improvement in intrahepatic lipid deposits using low doses of levothyroxine in euthyroid male patients with NAFLD and type 2 diabetes mellitus was shown to be beneficial in a trial. Small human studies including up to 40 patients with metabolic syndrome treated with T2 showed it may also be of some help. The use of T2 is experimental.

Thyroid hormone is an important signaling molecule to maintain normal metabolism, and studies have shown that regulation of the 3,5,3'-triiodothyronine (T3)/ thyroid hormone receptor axis is beneficial not only for metabolic symptoms but also for the improvement of NAFLD and even for the repair of liver injury. However, the non-selective regulation of T3 to thyroid receptor subtypes (TRα/TRβ) could cause unacceptable side effects represented by cardiotoxicity (heart toxicity). To avoid deleterious effects, TRβ-selective thyromimetics were developed for NASH studies in recent decades. Treatment with Resmetirom—a liver-directed, orally active, selective thyroid hormone receptor-B-agonist, in this class of drugs—resulted in significant reduction in hepatic fat after twelve weeks and thirty-six weeks of treatment in patients with NASH. Further studies of Resmetirom will allow assessment of safety and effectiveness of Resmetirom in a larger number of patients. It has been shown to improve NASH by increasing hepatic (liver) fat metabolism and reducing lipotoxicity, which is a metabolic syndrome that results from the accumulation of lipid intermediates in non-adipose tissue, leading to cellular dysfunction and death.

CONCLUSION

Nonalcoholic fatty liver disease (NAFLD) is the fastest-growing liver disease in the world. As you have seen, studies have shown that thyroid hormone replacement, in various forms, has been shown to be beneficial. Numerous other therapies, including LDN and nutritional therapies, along with the new drug Resmetirom, offer hope to patients with this common disease process. There is also evidence that the modification of mitochondrial function with nutritional support modulates NAFLD and that targeting the mitochondria is a promising new avenue for drug development to treat NAFLD/NASH.

13

Thyroid Hormones and Kidney Disease

growing body of evidence suggests that hypothyroidism is a risk factor for chronic kidney disease (CKD), CKD progression, and higher death risk in kidney disease patients. Various thyroid test abnormalities are frequently seen in CKD patients, resulting from alterations in thyroid hormone synthesis, metabolism, and regulation. Hyperthyroidism can also negatively impact kidney function.

KIDNEY FUNCTION TESTS

Your healthcare provider may order one or a few different types of kidney function tests. You may have blood tests for kidney function, such as:

- **Blood urea nitrogen (BUN)** measures nitrogen (made from protein breakdown) in your blood.

- **Estimated GFR (eGFR)** calculates filtration rates based on your protein levels, age, gender, size, and race.

- **Serum creatinine** looks for the buildup of creatinine, a waste product from muscle tissue breakdown.

Your healthcare provider may also order urine tests, including:

- **Urinalysis** evaluates your urine for blood, proteins, and function. Microalbumin is a blood protein filtered by the kidneys. The urine test measures the amount of this protein unfiltered by the kidneys and is used to detect early signs of kidney damage. A microalbumin level of 30 to 300 milligrams indicates early kidney disease, and more than 300 milligrams indicates advanced kidney disease.

THYROID DISORDERS AND KIDNEY FUNCTION

Thyroid dysfunction affects renal blood flow, glomerular filtration rate, (a blood test that measures how much blood your kidneys filter each minute) tubular function, electrolyte balance, and kidney structure. The various effects of hypothyroidism and hyperthyroidism on kidney function are summarized below.

Hypothyroidism and Kidney Function

If you have hypothyroidism, the following are possible negative influences that can occur related to your kidney and associated organs:

- Decreased heart rate
- Decreased cardiac (heart) contractility
- Decreased cardiac output
- Increased peripheral vascular resistance
- Decreased renal blood flow
- Decreased B-adrenergic receptors in the kidneys
- Decreased renin-angiotensin-aldosterone (RAAS) activity—regulator of blood volume, electrolyte balance, and systemic vascular resistance (SVR)
- Decreased filtration pressure
- Decreased glomerular filtration rate (GFR). The GFR is reversibly reduced by

- about 4 percent in more than 55 percent of adults with hypothyroidism
- Decreased tubuloglomerular feedback (a mechanism the kidney uses to regulate GFR)
- Decreased tubular mass
- Decreased NA/K ATPase
- Decreased NHE activity (red blood cell Na+/H+ exchange activity)
- Decreased urinary concentrating ability
- Hyponatremia (low sodium level) is twice as common among hypothyroid patients with raised serum creatinine as among those with normal serum creatinine

Hyperthyroidism and Kidney Function

If you have hyperthyroidism, the following are possible negative impacts that can occur related to your kidney and associated organs.

- Increased heart rate
- Increased cardiac (heart) contractility
- Increased cardiac output
- Decreased peripheral vascular resistance (PVR)
- Increased renal blood flow
- Increased B-adrenergic receptors in the kidneys
- Increased renin-angiotensin-aldosterone system (RAAS) activity
- Increased filtration pressure
- Increased glomerular filtration rate (GFR). The GFR increased by about 18 percent to 25 percent in hyperthyroid individuals in one study
- Increased tubuloglomerular feedback
- Increased tubular mass
- Increased NA/K ATPase
- Increased NHE activity (red blood cell Na+/H+ exchange activity)
- Decreased urinary concentrating ability

The great news is that with treatment of hypothyroidism or hyperthyroidism, your renal function commonly improves and/or normalizes.

CHRONIC KIDNEY DISEASE AND THYROID DYSFUNCTION

The reverse may also be true. Chronic kidney disease may be a risk factor for thyroid dysfunction.

Hypothyroidism and Chronic Kidney Disease

Primary hypothyroidism (non-autoimmune) is commonly observed in individuals with chronic kidney disease. In fact, the prevalence of subclinical hypothyroidism increases consistently with decline in kidney function. One study showed that approximately 18 percent of the patients with CKD not requiring dialysis have subclinical primary hypothyroidism. This finding was independently associated with a progressively lower estimated GFR.

Low thyroid hormones, especially low triiodothyronine levels free (T3), in patients with chronic kidney disease have been shown to be related to a higher risk of cardiovascular disease and all-cause mortality. Moreover, chronic kidney disease results in reduced iodide excretion, which results in increased serum inorganic iodide level and the thyroid gland iodine content and consequent thyroid gland enlargement. In addition, structural changes in the thyroid among chronic kidney disease patients include an increased prevalence of goiter (especially among women), thyroid nodules, and thyroid carcinoma, compared to general population. Interestingly, there is no increase in the incidence of autoimmune thyroid disease in CKD patients. In fact, the incidence of positive thyroglobulin and thyroid microsomal antibodies is low in chronic kidney disease individuals. However, autoimmune thyroid disease may occur along with other autoimmune diseases associated with CKD, such as lupus nephritis, type 1 diabetes mellitus, and others.

When elevated TSH is detected in association with other autoimmune diseases, it is important to have your healthcare provider screen for antithyroid antibodies. Treatment of hypothyroidism can result in improvement of kidney function (GFR) in chronic kidney disease individuals. In fact, in a clinical trial, subjects that were given thyroid medication had a slower rate of decline in kidney function and were less likely to develop end-stage kidney disease.

Hyperthyroidism and Chronic Kidney Disease

The prevalence of hyperthyroidism in CKD patients is the same as it is with the general population; thus, chronic kidney disease is not directly associated with hyperthyroidism. However, it is important to understand that hyperthyroidism can result in and accelerate chronic kidney disease by several mechanisms.

- Increased renal blood flow seen in hyperthyroidism results in intraglomerular (specialized cells located among the glomerular capillaries within the kidney) hypertension, leading to increased filtration pressure and consequent hyperfiltration. Proteinuria (high level of protein in urine) seen in hyperthyroidism is known to cause direct renal (kidney) injury.

- Increased mitochondrial energy metabolism along with downregulation of superoxide dismutase (antioxidant defense against oxidative stress in the body), which occurs in hyperthyroidism, contributes to an increased free radical generation that causes kidney injury.

- Oxidative stress also contributes to hypertension in hyperthyroidism, which contributes to CKD progression.

Two Large Studies on Thyroid Disorders and Kidney Disease

In a cross-sectional analysis of over 400,000 U.S. veterans who underwent repeated measures of serum TSH and kidney function tests (BUN, creatinine, and GFR), a decrease in GFR was associated with a higher risk of hypothyroidism, independent of socio-demographics, and comorbidities (distinct health conditions that are present at the same time).

Another study revealed the same association between thyroid disease and kidney disease. A prospective cohort study of 104,633 South Korean patients from the Kangbuk Samsung Health Study revealed that people with the highest TSH had a higher risk of developing chronic kidney disease.

CONCLUSION

Thyroid hormones influence renal development, kidney structure, renal hemodynamics (flow of blood within organs and tissues), GFR, the function of many transport systems along the nephron, and sodium and water balance. These effects of thyroid hormone are in part due to direct renal actions and in part are mediated by cardiovascular and systemic hemodynamic (related to the flow of blood) effects that influence kidney function. As a result, both hypothyroidism and hyperthyroidism are associated with clinically important changes in kidney function and have relevance to its assessment. Disorders of thyroid function have also been linked to development of immune-mediated glomerular injury, and alterations in thyroid hormones and thyroid hormone lab work can occur in individuals with kidney disease.

The impacts of hypothyroidism on the kidney are usually opposite to the effects one would see in hyperthyroidism. Fortunately, most of the renal manifestations of thyroid disease are reversible with treatment of the thyroid dysfunction. Moreover, more studies are needed to determine the impact of thyroid hormone replacement upon kidney disease progression, cardiovascular disease, and mortality, which may shed light onto the causal implications of both hypothyroidism and hyperthyroidism in chronic kidney disease.

14

Reproductive System and Thyroid Hormones: Women and Men

Your body is a holistic system. Nothing happens in isolation. It's not surprising that when one hormone is out of balance, it affects other hormones as well, particularly since your thyroid regulates many of the hormones in your body.

There is a great deal of scientific evidence recognizing that thyroid hormones are related to many aspects of human metabolism. Therefore, thyroid hormones should be monitored in both women and men and in people of all age groups. Both hypothyroidism and hyperthyroidism influence the metabolism of sex steroids. Consequently, without optimal function of both T3 and T4; estrogen, progesterone, testosterone, DHEA, cortisol, and pregnenolone will not perform adequately in your body no matter what sex you are. This phenomenon can precede to not just symptoms of hormonal dysregulation, but also can lead to an increased risk of developing major diseases such as infertility, polycystic ovarian disease (PCOS), heart disease, osteoporosis, and cognitive decline. Your hormone levels even affect the youthfulness of your skin.

It is paramount that you see a healthcare provider trained in Anti-Aging Medicine/Personalized Medicine or your compounding pharmacist to have your sex hormone levels measured by saliva testing. Pregnenolone is a blood study.

THYROID HORMONES AND WOMEN'S HORMONES

Thyroid hormones are vital for the proper functioning of the female reproductive system, since they modulate the metabolism and development of ovarian, uterine, and placental tissues. Therefore, hypo- and hyperthyroidism may result in subfertility or infertility in women. Infertility is also common in women with Graves' disease and Hashimoto's thyroiditis, affecting about 50 percent of people. Other well-documented sequelae (complications that result from pre-existing conditions) of maternal thyroid dysfunctions include, anovulation, miscarriage, preterm delivery, preeclampsia (high blood pressure during pregnancy with an increase of protein in the urine), intrauterine growth restriction, and postpartum thyroiditis.

Likewise, both hyper- and hypothyroidism may result in menstrual disturbances. The menstrual cycle is governed by a network of gonadotropins, which secrete hormones. For example, luteinizing hormone (LH) and follicle-stimulating hormone (FSH)) and sex steroid hormones (such as, estrogens and progesterone); key constituents of the hypothalamic-pituitary-gonadal axis. This system is closely related to the hypothalamic-pituitary-thyroid axis, which controls thyroid function. However, the relationship between thyroid function and female reproductive physiology is complex. Women are more likely to develop thyroid disease than men, and the incidence is greatest during times of hormonal flux, such as menopause, puberty, and pregnancy.

One study looked at the prevalence of menstrual disturbances, including secondary amenorrhea (abnormal absence of menstruation), hypomenorrhea (short or scanty periods), oligomenorrhea (less frequent periods where you may regularly go for more than 35 days between periods), hypermenorrhea (called menorrhagia, which is abnormally heavy bleeding during menstruation), and polymenorrhea (cycle occurs more commonly than every 21 days) were prospectively examined in 586 patients with hyperthyroidism due to Graves' disease, 111 with hypothyroidism, 558 with euthyroid chronic thyroiditis, 202 with painless thyroiditis, and 595 with thyroid tumor. In the overall patient group, the prevalence was not different from that in 105 healthy controls. However, patients with severe hyperthyroidism showed a higher prevalence of secondary amenorrhea and hypomenorrhea than those with mild or moderate hyperthyroidism. Moreover, patients with severe hypothyroidism had a higher prevalence (34.8 percent) of menstrual disturbances than mild-moderate cases (10.2 percent). Interestingly, menstrual disturbances in thyroid dysfunction were less frequent than previously thought since people were being diagnosed with thyroid disorders sooner in their disease continuum.

Another trial revealed that 30 percent of patients that had dysfunctional uterine bleeding (DUB) had thyroid dysfunction. Dysfunctional uterine bleeding is abnormal uterine bleeding between monthly periods, prolonged bleeding, or an extremely heavy period. Of those, 18 percent had subclinical hypothyroidism, 9 percent had polymenorrhagia, and 3 percent of hyperthyroid patients had oligomenorrhagia. In hyperthyroidism, the most common manifestation was simple oligomenorrhea (decreased menstrual flow). Anovulatory cycles (menstrual cycle in, which ovulation does not occur) were very common. Increased bleeding may also occur, but it is rare.

Fertility has been shown to be reduced in both hyper- and hypothyroidism, and the outcome of pregnancy is more often abnormal than in women with optimal thyroid function.

Galactorrhea (excessive production of breast milk) may also be present in hypothyroidism, possibly because TSH, the hypophyseal TSH-releasing hormone, increases the secretion of both TSH and prolactin, which is the hormone that is responsible for lactation.

In addition, ovarian volumes of individuals with hypothyroidism were significantly greater compared with controls, and their magnitudes diminished significantly during thyroid hormone replacement therapy. Women with hypothyroidism with polycystic ovaries (PCOS) had significantly higher serum free testosterone and dehydroepiandrosterone-sulfate (DHEA-S), but lower androstenedione (steroid hormone) levels compared with those who had normal-appearing ovaries. Therefore, severe long-standing hypothyroidism may lead to increased ovarian volume and/or cyst formation. Furthermore, a decrease in ovarian volume, resolution of ovarian cysts, and reversal of the polycystic ovary syndrome-like appearance, together with improvement in serum hormone levels, occurred after optimal thyroid function was achieved in a clinical trial. Moreover, serum total testosterone concentrations were significantly higher in individuals with hypothyroidism without polycystic ovaries, and thyroid hormone replacement therapy achieved a significant reduction in total as well as free testosterone to normal levels.

THYROID HORMONES AND MALE HORMONES

Previously, the thyroid gland was presumed not to have any impact on spermatogenesis—sperm cell production—and male fertility, however, it is now being recognized as having an important role in male reproductive functions. Both hypo- and hyperthyroidism can negatively impact male hormones as well as sex hormone-binding hormonal globulin (SHBG) concentrations. Sex hormone binding globulin is a hormone that binds and carries sex hormones, such as testosterone and estrogen (yes men make estrogen), to the tissue and organs where they are needed.

Men with hyperthyroidism have elevated concentrations of testosterone and SHBG. In addition, estradiol (a kind of estrogen) elevations are observed in men with hyperthyroidism, and gynecomastia is common in them as well. Gynecomastia is an increase in the amount of breast tissue in boys or men caused by an imbalance of the hormones estrogen and testosterone. Conversely, hypothyroidism has been shown to be associated with a reduction in serum testosterone level in males. This reduction in testosterone is reversible by thyroid hormone replacement.

CONCLUSION

As you have seen, both hyperthyroidism and hypothyroidism can impact the sex hormones of both men and women and cause changes in fertility and other major functions in the body that are regulated by the sex hormones. See your healthcare provider or pharmacist to have your complete thyroid studies done as well as a saliva test of your sex hormones: estrogen, progesterone, testosterone, and DHEA. It is also important to have cortisol (your stress hormone) measured by saliva since it balances DHEA in your body.

15

Hypothyroidism and Weight Gain

The obesity epidemic is a major threat to health in most countries. There is an intimate relationship between weight gain/obesity and hypothyroidism. This chapter will explore three ideas related to this relationship. Firstly, weight gain may be due to hypothyroidism since thyroid hormones regulate basal metabolism. TSH levels are commonly at the upper limit of the normal range or slightly increased in obese children, adolescents, and adults and are positively correlated with an increase in body mass index (BMI). Second, abnormal thyroid function may be due to obesity. Low free T4 with a moderate increase in T3 or free T3 levels has been reported in obese individuals. Third, obesity may be related to an autoimmune process occurring in the thyroid gland.

The relationship between thyroid function and weight is so intricate that if you are taking thyroid medication, if you gain or lose 20 pounds, make sure you contact your healthcare provider since you may need a change in thyroid dose.

HYPOTHYROIDISM DIRECTLY TIED TO WEIGHT GAIN

Body composition and thyroid hormones appear to be closely related. Thyroid hormones regulate your metabolism including your basal metabolic rate. It plays an important role in glucose metabolism, food intake, and fat oxidation. In addition, thyroid dysfunction is associated with changes in body weight and composition, body temperature, and total and resting energy expenditure independent of physical activity. Therefore, hypothyroidism may be the hidden cause of a weight problem. Thyroid hormones can have a major effect on your waistline. Low thyroid function can add pounds to your body while making it difficult to lose weight.

This means that even if you watch what you eat, your body is less able to convert calories into energy. The calories that are not used up cause you to gain weight. Slowly, over time, you can gain 5 to 15 pounds without even realizing it. Furthermore, the combination of reduced metabolism and other symptoms of hypothyroidism makes losing weight very difficult. In fact, evidence suggests that even slight changes in thyroid function can contribute to the tendency to gain weight.

In addition, the depression and insomnia so often caused by hypothyroidism increase your likelihood of indulging in foods that are high in less desirous carbohydrates and "bad" fats. Likewise, the fatigue associated with an underactive thyroid makes it harder for you to engage in the physical activity necessary to burn extra calories. There is a great deal of clinical evidence that suggests that even mild or subclinical hypothyroidism is linked to weight gain and obesity.

There are several ways that you can improve thyroid function. One study revealed that even simple changes of lifestyle, characterized by increased physical activity and improvement in body composition without concomitant—occurring or existing—changes of BMI can lead to a decrease in TSH. In addition, another study showed that modification in body composition reduced inflammation, decreased the secretion of cytokines, and subsequent worsening of thyroid function. This phenomenon is not surprising since weight gain causes an inflammatory process in your body and when you lose weight you literally decrease inflammation.

As discussed earlier in this book, an optimal iodine level is needed to have perfect thyroid function. Contact your healthcare provider or pharmacist to have your iodine level measured. It is best measured as a first morning urine test. If your level is low, and if you take iodine, it may improve your thyroid function. It is important to re-measure iodine levels in 90 days since iodine can be toxic to the body if levels are elevated. Of course, your healthcare provider may also prescribe you thyroid medication if your thyroid function is suboptimal or low.

ABNORMAL THYROID FUNCTION DUE TO OBESITY

A new concept being examined in medical literature is that changes in TSH may actually be secondary to obesity itself. At present, it is unclear if the slight elevation of TSH values frequently present in obesity causes weight gain or if it is due to obesity induced activation of the hypothalamus-pituitary-thyroid (HPT) axis, causing an increase in serum TSH. In support of the later concept, these alterations seem to be a consequence, rather than a cause, of obesity since weight loss leads to a normalization of elevated thyroid hormone levels.

In this context, recent research has shown that being overweight can influence the function of the thyroid gland, usually leading to increased TSH concentrations and changes in the ratio between the hormones T3 and T4, though within the normal range. The cause of these changes is still unclear. However, several mechanisms have been proposed, including the adaptive process to increase energy expenditure, high leptin (high leptin contributes to increased likelihood of developing heart disease, diabetes, cancer, degenerative joint disease, surgical complications, and autoimmune disorders), changes in the activity of deiodinases, the presence of thyroid hormone resistance (a syndrome in, which the thyroid hormone levels are elevated but the TSH level is not suppressed, or not completely suppressed as would be expected, which essentially is when the thyroid gland does not response appropriately to thyroid hormone), chronic low-grade inflammation, and insulin resistance. Studies suggest that these changes in the thyroid function of obese individuals may contribute to the worsening of metabolic complications and the development of thyroid dysfunction.

OBESITY RELATED AUTOIMMUNE PROCESS

The link between obesity and the risk of autoimmune thyroid dysfunction, which is the main cause of hypothyroidism in adults, is an area in medicine under discussion. The prevalence of autoimmune thyroid disease in obesity has been reported to be 12.4 percent in children and between 10 percent and 60 percent in adults. Another trial addressed the interesting idea of a link between obesity, leptin, autoimmunity, and hypothyroidism. This study suggested that obesity is a risk factor for thyroid autoimmune disease, therefore suggesting a link between Hashimoto's thyroiditis and obesity.

CONCLUSION

As you have seen, your weight is regulated by thyroid function through three important processes. Weight gain may occur as a consequence of hypothyroidism. In addition, abnormal thyroid function may be due to obesity, and obesity may be related to an autoimmune process occurring in the thyroid gland.

16

Thyroid Hormone and Insulin Resistance

hyroid hormones have a significant effect on glucose (carbohydrate) metabolism and if a person develops insulin resistance. Insulin resistance indicates that the body has become resistant to the effects of insulin. The presence of disorders of carbohydrate metabolism have been demonstrated in thyroid disease involving both hyperthyroidism and hypothyroidism. The severity of the disease is proportional to the severity of these disorders. The possible influence of subclinical forms of both hyperthyroidism and hypothyroidism on carbohydrate disorders is still being explored. In hyperthyroidism, impaired glucose tolerance may be the result of mainly hepatic (liver) insulin resistance, whereas in hypothyroidism there is a decreased net extraction of glucose and blood flow after a meal in hypothyroid muscles and tissues. In other words, hypothyroid individuals have impairment in the ability of insulin to boost blood flow to the hypothyroidism-affected tissues. Importantly, the prevalence of thyroid disease in patients with diabetes is significantly higher than that in the general population. This indicates a possible interplay between thyroid status and insulin sensitivity.

INSULIN

Insulin is the hormone responsible for the regulation of blood sugar. Specifically, it regulates the metabolism of carbohydrates, fats, and protein by promoting the absorption of glucose from the blood into liver, fat, and skeletal muscle cells. Insulin is produced in the body with peak functioning of the pancreas along with optimal balancing of other hormones. Perfect insulin levels are a key to the best health possible. Insulin levels that are too high or too low can cause symptoms and increase the risk of developing several diseases.

Functions of Insulin

- Affects glycogen metabolism by stimulation of glycogen synthesis
- Aids other nutrients to get inside cells
- Counters the actions of adrenaline and cortisol in the body
- Has an anti-inflammatory effect on endothelial cells and macrophages
- Helps convert blood sugar into triglycerides
- Helps the body repair itself
- Increases expression of some lipogenic enzymes
- Keeps blood glucose levels from rising above optimal levels
- Partially regulates protein turnover rate
- Plays a major role in the production of serotonin
- Stimulates the development of muscle (but at high levels it turns off the production of muscle and increases the production of fat)
- Suppresses reactive oxygen species (ROS)

Have your healthcare provider measure your fasting insulin level. Fasting serum insulin is used as an index of insulin sensitivity and resistance. The optimal fasting insulin level is 6 uIU/mL. Insulin levels that are too low or too high signify that insulin is not working optimally in your body. Commonly your doctor will measure your fasting blood sugar (FBS) and maybe also your hemoglobin A1c. Your hemoglobin A1c test is your average level of blood sugar over the past two to three months. It's also called HbA1c, glycated hemoglobin test, and glycohemoglobin. It is rare unless you see a practitioner that specializes in Personalized/Anti-Aging Medicine that you would have your fasting insulin level measured. Make sure you request this test from your doctor.

Signs and Symptoms of Insulin Deficiency

- Blurred vision
- Bone loss
- Confusion
- Depression

- Dizziness
- Fainting
- Fatigue
- Hunger
- Hypoglycemia
- Insomnia

- Insulin resistance
- Loss of consciousness (late stage)
- Palpitations
- Seizures (late stage)
- Sweating

Causes of Insulin Deficiency

- Eliminating carbohydrates from the diet
- Hypopituitarism
- Insulin resistance/diabetes
- Not eating enough
- Over-exercising without sufficient food and nutritional support
- Pancreatic diseases, such as chronic pancreatitis, cancer of the pancreas, and cystic fibrosis

Conditions Associated with Low Insulin Production

- Depression and mood swings
- Fatigue
- Insomnia

- Insulin resistance/diabetes
- Osteopenia/osteoporosis

When you eat complex carbohydrates and simple sugars, your insulin levels climb. If you eat too much sugar, your body produces more and more insulin until the insulin level is elevated and it does not work as effectively as it should. The medical term for this is insulin resistance.

Insulin is part of the hormonal symphony in your body, so when it is not performing optimally, all the other hormones are affected. Your body will attempt to compensate for insulin's decreased effects by producing more and more insulin. This can result in high insulin levels all the time, which can cause the cells in your adrenal glands, called theca cells, to turn on an enzyme called 17, 20-lyase. This enzyme causes your body's hormones to stop making estrogens and instead make androgens. (Both estrogens and androgens are made from DHEA.) This shift in hormonal balance can cause you to gain weight around the middle. It may also promote further insulin resistance. In fact, prolonged levels of high insulin can lead to diabetes. Furthermore, most major processes that lead to hardening of the arteries are caused by the overproduction of insulin as are some forms of memory loss. High insulin levels may also contribute to an increase in breast cancer risk.

When you eat simple sugars and consume caffeine to help with fatigue, not only will your adrenal glands suffer, but this will contribute to an elevated level of insulin in your body. Additionally, this causes your body to produce gas and you may experience bloating. Water is pulled into your colon from the bloodstream to respond to the high sugar load, which can lead to lose stools. Furthermore, you may develop gluten sensitivity from overeating carbohydrates.

There are many habits that can elevate insulin besides eating a diet high in simple sugars. Having a lot of stress, which causes your cortisol levels to be abnormal, will have a negative impact on insulin production. The following list contains lifestyle choices that raise insulin, as per Dr. Diana Schwarzbein, an endocrinologist and author of *The Schwarzbein Principle* and *The Schwarzbein Principle II*.

Causes of Excess Insulin Production

- Cigarette smoking
- Consuming soft drinks
- Eating a low-fat diet
- Eating trans-fat (partially hydrogenated or hydrogenated)
- Elevated DHEA levels
- Excessive alcohol consumption
- Excessive caffeine intake
- Excessive or unnecessary thyroid hormone replacement
- Excessive progesterone replacement
- Increased testosterone levels (male or female)
- Lack of exercise
- Poor sleep hygiene
- Skipping meals
- Some over-the-counter cold medications (any that contain caffeine)
- Some prescription medications (these are the most common)
- Beta-blockers
- Levodopa
- Oral contraceptives

- Some medications for depression and psychosis
- Steroids
- Thiazide diuretics
- Stress
- Taking diet pills

- Taking thyroid hormone replacement while not eating enough
- Use of artificial sweeteners
- Use of natural stimulants
- Use of recreational stimulants
- Yo-yo dieting

Elevated insulin levels can be lowered by eating a balanced diet of carbohydrates, proteins, and fats. The right amount of exercise (three or four times a week) can help to normalize insulin levels. Changing medications, quitting smoking, discontinuing stimulants, and decreasing or stopping caffeine consumption can also be beneficial. In addition, there are nutrients that can help insulin work more effectively in the body. Alpha lipoic acid, chromium, and vitamin D all do just this. However, these supplements can be very powerful, so if you are already taking a drug that lowers your blood sugar, you may need less medication with the use of these products. Make sure you monitor your blood sugar closely. Moreover, alpha lipoic acid has even been shown to prevent and treat diabetic neuropathy, a condition in, which the body's nerves become damaged due to diabetes. (See "Insulin Resistance" on page 284 for further information.)

Conditions Associated With Excess Insulin Production

- Acceleration of aging
- Acne
- Acromegaly (when your body makes too much growth hormone)
- Asthma
- Cushing's syndrome
- Depression and mood swings
- Estrogen levels that are too low
- Heart disease

- Heartburn
- Hypercholesterolemia
- Hypertension
- Hypertriglyceridemia
- Increased risk of developing cancer
- Infertility
- Insomnia
- Insulin resistance/diabetes
- Irritable bowel syndrome

- Metabolic syndrome
- Migraine headaches
- Osteopenia/osteoporosis
- Weight gain

INSULIN RESISTANCE

Insulin resistance is defined as a glucose homeostasis disorder involving a decreased sensitivity of muscles, adipose tissue, liver, and other body tissues to insulin, despite its normal or increased concentration in blood. Therefore, insulin resistance is evident when cells do not properly absorb glucose, the body's preferred source of fuel, resulting in a buildup in the blood. Consequently, insulin resistance occurs when insulin is present but does not work as effectively in the body as it should. Therefore, levels start to rise to help the body compensate for less than effective insulin function. Insulin resistance may be asymptomatic or occur presenting a variety of disorders, such as: glucose tolerance impairment, type 2 diabetes, as well as hypercholesterolemia (high cholesterol), hypertriglyceridemia (high triglycerides), obesity, and arterial hypertension (high blood pressure).

More than 80 percent of the adult population in the United States has blood glucose levels that are too high. If a patient has a fasting blood sugar (FBS) that is high-normal (over 85 mg/dL), the risk of the patient dying of cardiovascular disease (heart disease) is increased by 40 percent. Furthermore, having a FBS that is high-normal increases your risk of vascular death. Insulin also plays a profound role in cognitive function. High-normal levels of FBS may account for a decrease in the volume of the hippocampus and amygdala of 6 to 10 percent. Consequently, insulin resistance is a risk factor for cognitive decline. Also, the "Honolulu-Asia Aging Study" showed that the effect of hyperinsulinemia (high insulin levels) on the risk of dementia was independent of diabetes and blood glucose. Therefore, growing evidence supports the concept that insulin resistance is important in the pathogenesis of cognitive impairment and neurodegeneration.

Sign and Symptoms of Insulin Resistance

- Fuzzy brain
- Infertility
- Irregular menstrual cycles
- Irritability
- Loose bowel movements alternating with constipation
- Water retention
- Weight gain

Causes of Insulin Resistance

Insulin resistance has many possible causes. Here are some reasons why individuals with insulin resistance are not able to effectively use insulin.

- Abuse of alcohol
- Decreased estrogen levels
- Eating processed foods
- Elevated DHEA levels
- Excessive caffeine intake
- Excessive dieting
- Excessive progesterone in females (prescribed)
- Genetic susceptibility
- Hypothyroidism
- Increased stress
- Increased testosterone
- Insomnia
- Lack of exercise
- Use of nicotine
- Use of oral contraceptives

Conventional Treatments

Conventional treatments for insulin resistance involve exercise and a diet centered on consumption of foods with low glycemic index numbers. If an individual is overweight, then weight reduction is very beneficial. If these methods are not successful, then medications may be added.

While no medications are FDA approved for the treatment of insulin resistance, general approaches include the following, which are medications used for diabetes:

- **Metformin:** This is considered first-line therapy for medication treatment of type 2 diabetes and is approved for use in polycystic ovary syndrome. The DPP/DPPO study showed that the addition of metformin and lifestyle interventions combined were medically useful and cost-effective.

- **Glucagon-like peptide one inhibitors:** The GLP-1 receptor agonists stimulate the GLP-1 receptors in the pancreas, thereby increasing insulin release and inhibiting glucagon—hormone that controls glucose levels—secretion. Use of GLP-1 agonists are associated with weight loss, which may reduce insulin resistance. Liraglutide is FDA approved as an anti-obesity agent.

- **Sodium-glucose cotransporter two inhibitors:** The SGLT2 inhibitors increase the excretion of urinary glucose, thereby reducing plasma glucose levels and exogenous insulin requirements. Use of SGLT2 inhibitors has also been associated with weight loss, which may reduce insulin resistance.

- **Thiazolidinediones:** TZDs improve insulin sensitivity by increasing insulin-dependent glucose disposal in muscle and adipose tissue as well as decreasing hepatic glucose output. Though effective, associated secondary weight gain and fluid retention, with associated cardiovascular concerns, limit their use.

- **Dipeptidyl peptidase-4 inhibitors:** Dipeptidyl peptidase 4 (DPP-4) inhibition prevents the rapid degradation of the incretins, glucagon-like peptide 1 and glucose-dependent insulinotropic peptide. Incretins have beneficial effects on glycemic control in patients with type 2 diabetes through their effects on both alpha- and beta-cells in the pancreas and possibly through additional non-pancreatic effects.

Personalized/Anti-Aging Medicine Therapies

Personalized/Anti-Aging Medicine has many therapies to improve and sometimes even reverse insulin resistance.

Exercise

The first one is exercise. Lack of exercise is a risk factor for the development of insulin resistance and diabetes in susceptible individuals. Exercising four days a week for an hour a day has been shown to be beneficial. If you are over the age of 40 and have not been exercising, then see your healthcare provider for an evaluation before you begin an exercise program.

Diet

Eating foods that are low on the glycemic index (GI) is important. The GI ranks carbohydrate-containing foods on a scale from 0 to 100 according to the speed with, which they enter the bloodstream and raise glucose levels. Foods high on the list increase blood sugar and cause insulin to rise. One study showed that insulin secretion was lower in people who were on a low glycemic index program for only two weeks. The glycemic index is affected by the size of the particles into, which the food breaks down. Therefore, the more the processed the food or the longer it is cooked, the higher its glycemic index. The best carbohydrates that curb insulin are broccoli, lentils, and chickpeas. In addition, the fat content of a food influences its glycemic index ranking. Fat slows down sugar absorption and therefore lowers the glycemic index number.

The right balance of saturated to polyunsaturated to monounsaturated fats is important both for the prevention and treatment of insulin resistance and diabetes. Likewise, a high-fiber diet is crucial. Soluble fiber has been shown to lower insulin levels. Furthermore, getting enough protein in the diet decreases the absorption of sugars and consequently decreases your glycemic load. Weight loss has been shown to be helpful as well.

Good Sleep Hygiene

Moreover, getting a good night's sleep has been shown to be beneficial. If you do not sleep at least six and a half hours a night, then insulin levels may rise and lead to insulin resistance.

Optimal Thyroid Function

If you are hypo- or hyperthyroid, treating the disease has been shown to improve insulin resistance. If you are hypothyroid, or have subclinical hypothyroidism, insulin does not work optimally in your body. One study revealed that lower TSH and higher T4 levels in hypothyroid patients are associated with improved insulin sensitivity, higher HDL, and better endothelial (inner lining of blood vessels) function. In addition, it has long been recognized that hyperthyroidism promotes hyperglycemia (high blood sugar), which is a condition where insulin also does not work effectively in the body.

Hormone Replacement Therapy

In both men and women, optimal levels of the sex hormones have been shown to optimal blood sugar and insulin levels. These hormones include estrogen, progesterone, testosterone, DHEA, and cortisol. See an Anti-Aging/Personalized Medicine healthcare provider or a compounding pharmacist to have a saliva test done to have these hormones measured.

Nutrients

There are also many nutritional supplements and botanical nutrients that have clinical trials supporting their use in insulin resistance.

TABLE 16.1. SUPPLEMENTS TO TREAT INSULIN RESISTANCE

Supplements	Dosage	Considerations
Alpha lipoic acid	100 mg to 400 mg daily	Alpha lipoic acid improves blood sugar levels, so diabetics may be able to take less medication. Alpha lipoic acid also slows the development of diabetic neuropathy. Consult your healthcare provider if you are considering taking more than 500 mg in a day. Larger doses can negatively impact thyroid functioning.
Arginine	1,000 to 5,000 mg once a day	Do not take if you have kidney disease, liver disease, or herpes except under a doctor's supervision. Arginine can interact with some medications. Consult with your healthcare provider before beginning this therapy.
Asian ginseng*	50 to 200 mg of extract standardized to 4 percent ginsenosides twice a day	Always take with food. Use with caution if you have high blood pressure. Do not use if you are taking a blood thinner or if you have a hormonally related cancer such as breast, prostate, uterine, or ovarian.
B-complex vitamins	50 mg twice a day	I suggest taking a multivitamin along with your B-complex vitamins.
Berberine*	Start with 200 mg twice a day (You may go up to 500 mg three times a day)	Do not use this supplement during pregnancy. It can cause uterine contractions.
Bergamot	800 mg once or twice a day	It also blocks the rate-limiting step in cholesterol production. If you are on a cholesterol lowering medication, have your healthcare provider measure your cholesterol after three months. You may need a lower dose of the drug.
Carnitine*	2,000 to 3,000 mg once a day	Have your healthcare provider measure your TMAO levels before starting long-term supplementation with carnitine.
Carnosine	2,000 mg once a day	Check with your doctor before starting carnosine therapy if you have diabetes, hypertension, kidney disease, or liver damage. Too much carnosine can result in hyperactivity.

Chromium	300 to 1,000 mcg once a day as chromium picolinate	Combining with the protein picolinate allows your body to absorb chromium more efficiently. However, some chromium picolinate supplements contain more chromium than necessary. Ask your healthcare provider for a recommendation on chromium consumption.
Coenzyme Q-10*	30 to 200 mg daily	If you are on blood-thinning medications, speak to your healthcare provider before using CoQ-10. Since some medications can cause a deficiency of this nutrient, speak to your healthcare provider to determine if you might need a larger dose.
Copper	2 to 3 mg once a day	Your copper-to-zinc ratio is very important for your health. Also, do not take copper supplement cupric oxide, which has a very low bioavailability.
Cysteine	500 mg once a day as n-acetylcysteine, or NAC	When taking NAC supplements, also take extra vitamin C, copper, and zinc.
D-ribose	15,000 mg three times a day	D-ribose can lower blood sugar levels, so check with your healthcare provider before taking this supplement with any diabetes medication, especially insulin.
EPA/DHA (fish oil)*	1,000 to 2,000 mg once a day	Choose a source that contains vitamin E to prevent oxidation.
Fenugreek*	50 mg of seed powder twice a day, or 2 to 4.5 ml of 1:2 liquid extract twice a day	Avoid fenugreek if you are allergic to chickpeas, peanuts, green peas, or soybeans. Fenugreek has mild blood-thinning effects. If you have a bleeding disorder or are taking a medication or supplement that may thin your blood, do not take this herb. Fenugreek may also negatively impact thyroid functioning.
Fiber, soluble	Suggested daily intake is 25 grams for women and 38 grams for men (Try to get most of your fiber from whole foods)	Choose a fiber supplement with no added sugar, and take with several glasses of water to prevent side effects.
Ginkgo biloba*	120 mg once daily	Do not use with blood-thinning medications or supplements.

Green coffee bean extract	400 mg a day	Because green coffee contains caffeine, you should avoid taking this supplement if you are sensitive to caffeine.
Gymnema sylvestre	400 to 600 mg a day of an extract that contains 24 percent gymnemic acid	Stop taking this supplement two weeks before surgery, as it can interfere with blood sugar control during and after surgical procedures. At high doses, gymnema can cause gastric irritation or liver toxicity.
Inositol	2,000 to 4,000 mg once a day	May stimulate uterine contractions. Women who wish to become pregnant should consult their doctor regarding its use. Doses larger than 200 mg should be taken only under physician supervision.
Magnesium	400 to 800 mg once a day	Consult your healthcare provider for dosage if you have kidney disease. Discontinue use and see your doctor if you experience abdominal pain. Take a lower dose if it causes diarrhea.
Manganese	2 to 5 mg once a day	Use with caution if you have gallbladder or liver disease.
Olive leaf extract*	500 mg to 750 mg a day containing 20 mg of oleuropein per capsule	Olive leaf extracts can interact with many prescription medications, and may increase the effects of blood thinners. Consult your healthcare provider before using olive leaf extract if you are taking any medication. Don't use if you are pregnant or breastfeeding.
Quercetin*	300 mg three times a day	For best results, take with bromelain and vitamin C. Do not use with blood-thinning medications or supplements.
Selenium	200 mcg once a day	Do not exceed 200 mcg a day without consulting your healthcare provider.
Taurine	1,000 to 1,500 mg once a day	Take between meals. Discontinue use if you suddenly have feelings of chest or throat tightness or if you break out in hives. Do not take with aspirin. Have your healthcare provider measure levels before starting taurine therapy.
Vanadium*	50 mcg once a day	Do not take more than 50 mcg a day without a doctor's supervision. Do not use if you are taking blood-thinning medications or supplements.

Vitamin B$_6$ (pyridoxine)	75 mg twice a day	Do not take more than 500 mg a day. If you are taking L-dopa for Parkinson's disease, do not take B$_6$ without first consulting your doctor. High doses can deplete your body of other vitamins in the B complex, so take a B-complex vitamin twice a day.
Vitamin B$_7$ (biotin)	8 to 10 mg once a day	Large doses of biotin can deplete your body of other vitamins in the B complex, so take B-complex vitamins twice a day. Biotin can also negatively impact thyroid function.
Vitamin B$_{12}$ (cobalamin)	500 to 1,500 mcg twice a day	High doses can deplete your body of other vitamins in the B complex, so take with a B-complex vitamin twice a day.
Vitamin C	500 to 1,500 mg twice a day	Do not take high doses if you are prone to kidney stones or gout. High doses can also cause diarrhea.
Vitamin D$_3$	Have your blood levels measured by your healthcare provider, who will determine proper dosage	You can become vitamin D toxic. Therefore, have your healthcare provider measure your levels to determine the perfect dose for you.
Vitamin E*	400 to 800 IU once a day	Take mixed tocopherols, the more active type of vitamin E. Consult your healthcare provider first if you are taking a blood thinner.
Zinc	20 to 50 mg once a day as zinc picolinate or zinc citrate	Your copper-to-zinc ratio is very important to your health. If you are taking zinc and iron supplements, take one in the morning and one in the evening. (Taking them together reduces the efficiency of both.)

*This supplement can have a blood-thinning action.

As you have seen, it is important to have optimal levels of insulin in the body. Insulin, like many hormones, is regulated by your thyroid hormones. Therefore, optimal levels of T3 and T4 are needed in order for your body to produce the perfect level of insulin.

Therapeutic Benefits of Optimal Insulin Levels

- Helps to normalize weight
- Memory maintenance
- Prevention and treatment of insulin resistance and diabetes

- Prevention and treatment of polycystic ovary syndrome (PCOS)
- Prevention of coronary heart disease

- Prevention of hypertension
- Prevention of osteoporosis/ osteopenia
- Prevention of some cancers

CONCLUSION

Insulin resistance is identified as an impaired biologic response to insulin stimulation of target tissues, primarily the liver, muscle, and adipose tissue. Insulin resistance impairs glucose disposal, resulting in a compensatory increase in beta-cell insulin production and hyperinsulinemia (high insulin levels). The metabolic consequences of insulin resistance can result in hyperglycemia (high blood sugar), hypertension (high blood pressure), dyslipidemia (abnormal lipid levels), abdominal fat, hyperuricemia (high uric acid levels), elevated inflammatory markers, endothelial dysfunction (a type of coronary heart disease), and a prothrombic state (hypercoagulable state). Progression of insulin resistance can lead to metabolic syndrome, nonalcoholic fatty liver disease (NAFLD), and type 2 diabetes mellitus.

Many people in the United States, and the remainder of the world, have insulin resistance. The great news is that there are many therapies with proven clinical trials that have been shown to be effective in helping insulin to work more effectively in the body. One of these therapies is to treat thyroid dysfunction.

17

Thyroid Hormones and COVID-19/ Post-COVID Syndrome

COVID-19 has been shown to affect several organs and systems, including the endocrine system with possible short and long-term consequences. For instance, the pituitary-thyroid axis should be considered a susceptible target of SARS-CoV-2, and a direct or indirect pituitary injury has been described as a determining factor of possible secondary hypothyroidism. In line with these concepts, thyroid changes have been observed during and after a COVID-19 infection. In fact, around 15 percent of patients with mild to moderate COVID-19 had thyroid dysfunction.

More specifically, there has been a direct effect of SARS-CoV-2 on thyroid function in four different ways. First, potentially leading to exacerbation of pre-existing autoimmune thyroid disease; second, low free T3, which is associated with systemic inflammation and subsequent thyroiditis, thirdly hyperthyroidism, and lastly via long-haul COVID syndrome.

THYROID AUTOIMMUNITY AND COVID-19

Thyroid autoimmunity was certainly a pre-existing and possibly undiagnosed condition in some people, but SARS-CoV-2 has been shown to have exacerbated this condition in some individuals. Persistent hypothyroidism, mostly due to Hashimoto's thyroiditis, has been described in seven percent of severe acute respiratory syndrome coronavirus survivors and these data suggest that coronaviruses may have a potential for inducing long-term thyroid dysfunction.

LOW T3 SYNDROME/INFLAMMATION AND COVID-19

A pre-existing or new-onset thyroid hormone imbalance, such as the low T3 syndrome (most likely due to systemic inflammation), may be associated with the disease severity in COVID-19. In March 2020, the first case of subacute thyroiditis diagnosed in an 18-year-old woman was described. The patient was admitted to the hospital with typical signs and symptoms of viral thyroiditis occurring 15 days after a SARS-CoV-2–positive was diagnosed within the context of a mild COVID-19 case. Subsequently, several other cases have been reported worldwide. In these patients' subacute thyroiditis symptoms occurred 16 to 36 days after the resolution of COVID-19. A prompt response to oral prednisone returned optimal thyroid balance after a few weeks of treatment.

HYPERTHYROIDISM (THYROTOXICOSIS)

Patients with hyperthyroidism (subnormal TSH levels) in a study were compared to those with normal TSH levels in individuals with COVID-19. They had a more frequent fever (89 percent vs. 59 percent) and a lower SARS-Cov-2 cycle threshold value at polymerase chain reaction (technique for rapid amplification of a specific segment of DNA) suggesting a higher viral load. In another retrospective study among 50 confirmed hospitalized COVID-19 patients, more than half of them had transiently subnormal TSH levels, and those with lower TSH values had a worse prognosis. Thyrotoxicosis was associated with a more significant hospital stay and a higher in-hospital mortality rate. IL-6 level was inversely related to TSH levels, and consequently, thyrotoxicosis resulted in higher concentrations of IL-6, a marker of greater inflammation. Furthermore, in people with more severe disease, higher c-reactive protein levels were also seen revealing further inflammation.

LONG-HAUL COVID

Post-COVID syndrome, also known as long-haul COVID, refers to symptoms persisting for more than three weeks after the diagnosis of COVID-19. The incidence of post-COVID syndrome is estimated at 10 to 35 percent, while for hospitalized patients it may reach 85 percent. Fatigue is the most common symptom reported in 17.5 to 72 percent of post-COVID cases, followed by residual dyspnea (difficulty breathing) with an incidence ranging from 10 to 40 percent. Sleeping disorders, anxiety, and depression affect up to 26 percent of patients. Chest pain, changes in taste and smell, may affect up to 22 percent and 11 percent of patients, respectively. More than one third of patients with post-COVID syndrome have pre-existing comorbidities, hypertension and diabetes mellitus being the most common. Likewise, long-haul COVID is linked to dysregulation of the thyroid gland in some people through several mechanisms.

One journal article presented three cases of thyroid dysfunction: Hashimoto's thyroiditis, Graves' disease, and subacute thyroiditis, which developed a few weeks after resolution of acute phase of COVID-19 infection in people with no prior thyroid disease. Another study presented a case of thyroid storm due to long-haul COVID. Thyroid storm is a rare but severe and potentially life-threatening complication of hyperthyroidism that is characterized by a very high fever, fast and often irregular heartbeat, elevated blood pressure, vomiting, diarrhea, and agitation. Fortunately, only one case has been reported.

Moreover, hypothyroidism has been shown to be associated with prolonged COVID-19-induced loss of smell. SARS-CoV-2- induced smell dysfunction could be triggered by a direct viral insult of both the olfactory nerve and the thyroid gland. The absence or the slow recovery of olfaction (sense of smell) may be due to the viral-induced downregulation of thyroid function that may blunt the effects of thyroid hormones into the maturation and regeneration of olfactory neuronal cells especially in individuals with a history of thyroid dysfunction.

CONCLUSION

SARS-CoV-2 can lead to short-term and reversible thyroid dysfunction. It must be kept in mind that the use of steroids and heparin may affect thyroid hormone secretion and measurement, leading to possible misdiagnosis of thyroid dysfunction in severe cases of COVID-19. In addition, high-risk thyroid nodules require a fine needle aspiration without delay. Fortunately, in most patients that have changes in thyroid function, it is mild, and resolves without sequalae—an after effect. However, there are those individuals that will have abnormal thyroid levels after COVID-19 has resolved due to long-haul COVID, which may in itself be an autoimmune process.

18

Thyroid Cancer

The number of thyroid cancer cases have more than doubled since the early 1970s, and for women, it is the cancer with the fastest-growing number of new cases. As of 2015, the incidence of thyroid cancer was estimated to be 62,450 cases in the U.S. It currently stands as the fifth most common cancer in women. And like most other thyroid diseases, it occurs approximately 3 times more often in women than in men. While that may sound frightening, the overall odds of beating most thyroid cancers are in your favor. So, the more you know, the better prepared you will be to understand what it is, and how, in most cases, it can be successfully treated.

It is also important to point out that just finding a nodule on the thyroid gland does not mean the growth is malignant. Each year there are over 1.2 million patients who are diagnosed with thyroid nodules. Many of these nodules are ruled out as benign using an ultrasound scan. Of the 525,000 to 600,000 nodules that are biopsied every year, only 10 percent are found to be malignant.

Still, knowledge is power, so this chapter has been designed to provide you with not only an understanding of the most common terms related to thyroid cancer, but also an overview of the entire process. It begins by looking at what thyroid cancer is then examines the risk factors involved, its many signs and symptoms, and the tests used to determine if it is thyroid cancer. Once test results come back, there will be descriptive terms used that patients need to understand. Explained are the most common terms under the sections on visual characteristics of thyroid cancer cells, its stages, and the standard treatments available. This is followed by a discussion concerning each type of thyroid cancer. The chapter concludes with practical suggestions patients should consider when preparing for what's ahead of them.

WHAT IS THYROID CANCER?

As discussed in Chapter 1, the thyroid gland is composed of several types of cells. This includes the follicular cells, the parafollicular cells (C cells), and the endothelial cells. When a clump of cells unexpectedly begins to grow in the thyroid, they may be either benign (non-cancerous) or malignant (cancerous). Benign growths tend to grow slowly and stop at a certain point; malignant growths, on the other hand, contain cells that begin to multiply uncontrollably and can spread to nearby tissues as well as other parts of the body. Tumors that have spread to other parts of the body are called metastasis. It is important to know that some thyroid cancers may grow very slowly and go undetected for years.

The type of thyroid cancer that may occur is based on the specific thyroid cell that has become malignant. Therefore, quickly learning what type of thyroid cancer the tumor is composed of is very important, since the odds of success are based on the make-up of the thyroid cancer. It is also valuable to know that some thyroid tumors can be composed of more than one type of malignant thyroid cell as well as benign cells. The good news is that the overall 5-year survival rate of individuals with the most common thyroid cancer is 98 percent. You will learn more about the survival rates of various types of thyroid cancers as they are discussed.

Risk Factors

While anyone may be susceptible to developing thyroid cancer, there are those who may be at a higher risk based upon the following risk factors:

Family History. Certain genes can be passed on from one generation to the next, which can greatly increase the odds of developing thyroid cancer. It has been found that where there is a family history of precancerous polyps in the colon or goiters, the risk of papillary thyroid cancer increases. In addition, specific medullary thyroid cancer-prone genes can be passed on as well.

Radiation Exposure. During the 1950s, children were treated using radiation therapy for noncancerous conditions, such as enlarged thymus, acne, ringworm, or enlargement of the tonsils or adenoids. Currently, children who have had imaging tests such as x-rays and CT scans or have undergone certain radiation treatments may have a higher risk of developing thyroid cancer. Similar exposure by adults may also increase the odds of their having this disease. In addition, anyone who has been exposed to radiation from power plant accidents or nuclear fallout may also be at greater risk of developing thyroid cancer.

Age and Gender. While thyroid cancer can develop in people who are in their 20s and up, statistics indicate that women in their 40s and 50s are 3 times more likely to develop thyroid cancer than men. For men, they are at greater risk in their 60s and 70s.

Iodine Intake. A lack of iodine in one's diet can lead to enlargement of the thyroid and mental retardation in infants and children. In addition, low iodine intake can increase the odds of developing follicular cancer and papillary cancer (with radiation exposure). Usually, the standard western diet provides a sufficient level of iodine through intake of iodized salt and other foods. Studies have also shown that excessive iodine supplementation may be linked to an increase in developing thyroid cancer. Therefore, it is important to have your iodine levels measured. A first morning urine is the most accurate test.

Environmental Pollutants. Studies investigating cancer risk factors associated with environmental pollutants have provided fascinating results. Some industrialized food additives, such as nitrates from cured meat and some vegetables, can compete with iodine uptake, potentially altering thyroid function, and inducing thyroid cancer. Another study showed that above-average nitrate levels in drinking water resources are also associated with an increased risk of this disease. Moreover, environmental pollutants, which may act as either genotoxic or nongenotoxic carcinogens, such as asbestos, benzene, formaldehyde, pesticides, and many others, may increase the risk. Polybrominated diphenyl ethers (PBDEs) that are used in building materials, electronics, furnishings, motor vehicles, airplanes, plastics, and textiles may induce abnormal thyroid cell proliferation, favoring a precancerous state.

Race. Statistics indicated that Caucasian and Asian people are more likely to develop thyroid cancer, however, it is important to point out that no one group is exempt. For example, while the black population shows the lowest rates of thyroid cancer among any groups, the greatest rate of papillary thyroid cancer acceleration has been recorded in black females. Still, while statistics may show a person's level of risk may be on the high side, anyone can be at risk; it is important for you to become aware of the signs and symptoms of thyroid cancer.

Sign and Symptoms

A number of the physical warning signs of thyroid cancer can provide us with an opportunity to catch it in an early stage. The following are the most common symptoms:

- Swollen lymph nodes. Normally, a swollen lymph gland is a sign of infection; however, it may also be the site of a thyroid cancer tumor.

- Lump in the neck. A new lump appearing in front of the Adam's apple or to either side may be an indication.

- Pain in the throat or neck. Unexplained pain in the throat or neck may be due to an enlargement of the neck caused by swollen lymph nodes or a tumor pressing against the trachea (windpipe) or esophagus.

- Hoarseness. Changes in your voice or a persistent hoarseness may be due to pressure from an enlarged thyroid gland or a growth, which sits just beneath the larynx (voice box).

- Difficulty swallowing. Unexplained pain when swallowing food may be caused by an enlargement of the neck or a tumor pressing against the trachea, which sits above the esophagus.

- Trouble breathing. Breathing difficulty may be caused by an enlargement of the neck or a tumor pressing against the trachea, which sits above the esophagus.

- Wheezing. Unexplained wheezing may be caused by an enlargement of the neck or a tumor pressing against the trachea.

- Persistent cough. A cough that is not due to a cold may be caused by an enlargement of the neck or a tumor pushing against the larynx or trachea.

- If any of these warning signs appear, without any recent history of infections, it would be wise to see a physician immediately to determine the cause of the problem. A toothache, a sinus infection, or a benign growth can mimic the signs of a cancerous nodule. The great news is that the quicker the cause is found, the quicker the right treatment can be applied.

Unfortunately, there are times thyroid cancer progresses without any early symptoms. Instead, the only signs and symptoms to appear occur when the thyroid cancer tumors interfere with the thyroid's normal regulation of life functions—from problems with weight, to blood pressure, to heart rate. The underlying problem may only be discovered through a thorough physical examination by a doctor who can perform or recommend several possible tests.

Testing

If the initial signs indicate a possible thyroid problem, there are a number of tests healthcare providers may offer patients to determine if they have thyroid cancer, and if they do, what type of thyroid cancer it is. The most common are the following.

Thyroid Ultrasound

Sound waves are used to create a visual image of the thyroid. This is done when a small wand-like instrument is moved along the skin in front of the thyroid gland. The black and white image seen on a computer screen will show whether the node is composed of a solid mass of cells or a cyst containing blood or pus. If it is a solid node, further testing needs to be done to determine if the mass is benign or cancerous.

Fine Needle Aspiration (FNA)

If the node is found to be solid, a fine needle aspiration is taken. The skin above the node is numbed, and a thin needle is inserted into the node to remove cells and fluid for review. These samples are then sent to a laboratory where a pathologist examines them under a microscope to determine the exact nature of the cells. The pathologist writes up a report on his/her findings and sends back the report to the ordering doctor.

While the FNA is designed to determine if the cells are benign or cancerous, up to 30 percent of the FNA biopsy may be inconclusive. In many cases another FNA is taken, however due to the type of thyroid cancer it may be, the results may still be inconclusive. When this happens a blood test may be able to provide an answer. However, should it not, traditionally, surgery is the next step to determine if the node is benign or cancerous. However, a personalized genetic test has been developed to provide an answer based on the initial FNA biopsy, which can prevent unnecessary surgeries. (See Personalized Genetic Test below.)

Personalized Genetic Test

Beyond just testing for inherited thyroid cancer-prone genes, there are personalized genetic tests available, which may be able to rule out whether the cells taken from a FNA procedure are benign or malignant. Additionally, the test may determine how aggressive a BRAF (a genetic alteration) gene-based thyroid cancer cell may be. These tests are based upon molecular identification. The results of such tests can enable a surgeon to determine how extensive a surgery is needed or if one is required at all.

Blood Calcitonin Test

Calcitonin is a hormone produced by the parafollicular cells, also known as C-cell, found in the thyroid. It acts to reduce calcium found in the blood. When the amount of calcitonin in the blood is found to be high, it can indicate the presence of C-cell hyperplasia, a pre-cancerous stage, which may lead to medullary thyroid cancer. However, C-cell hyperplasia, in and of itself, is a benign condition. This blood test may be ordered when any of the risk factors described above are present.

Blood Carcinoembryonic Antigen (CEA) Test

People with thyroid cancer that has spread often have high blood levels of a protein called carcinoembryonic antigen (CEA). Tests for CEA can help monitor this cancer.

Radioiodine Thyroid Scan

Unlike the thyroid ultrasound, the thyroid scan requires a radioactive iodine tracer be swallowed or injected into the blood stream. The signals given off by the radiation can measure how much tracer is absorbed from the blood and the scan itself can show the location, shape, and size of the gland as well as nodules that may be located within the gland.

Computed Tomography (CT)

A CT scan is a computerized x-ray that shows a detailed cross-sectional image of the thyroid and its surrounding area. It requires that a contrast solution be swallowed or given through an IV line. The solution contains a dye that outlines the thyroid gland along with any mass and structure within the neck area.

Magnetic Resonance Imaging (MRI)

Just like the CT scan, the MRI scan shows a more detailed cross-section of the thyroid and its surrounding area. Instead of x-rays, it uses radio waves and magnets to create its images. A contrasting solution is injected in the blood stream and the dye outlines the thyroid gland along with any mass and structure within the neck area.

Positron Emission Tomography (PET) Scan

A PET scan can produce a three-dimensional image using gamma rays. A substance containing a radioactive form of sugar is injected into the blood stream. The radioactive sugar is quickly absorbed by tumors, which will show up in its images. While not as finely detailed as CT or MRI scans, PET scans can provide a full body image of possible cancer sites, particularly if your thyroid cancer is one that does not take up radioactive iodine. In this situation, the PET scan may be able to determine if the cancer has spread.

PATHOLOGICAL CHARACTERISTICS OF THYROID CANCER CELLS

As we will see, the different kinds of thyroid cancers stem from specific types of thyroid cells. There are a number of important terms that are associated with the way these cancer cells appear. These terms are commonly used in pathology reports to provide a physician with a detailed picture of the type of cells contained in a tumor.

Differentiated cancer cells. While some cancer cells may look and behave like normal cells, others may change their appearance. Under a microscope, all their internal structures are clearly identifiable. Like normal thyroid cells, they absorb iodine; however, unlike normal cells these cancer cells will grow unregulated and may spread.

Poorly differentiated cancer cells. Under a microscope, these cells may be missing certain internal structures, or their internal structures are malformed. In some cases, there are enough functioning structures within the cell to identify the type of thyroid cell it originates from. However, sometimes identifying the origin of these cells is difficult. In some cases, they may also lack the ability to absorb iodine.

Undifferentiated cancer cells. Although these cells may originate from a specific thyroid cell, they do not contain enough internal structures to be linked to a specific type of thyroid cell. And unlike other thyroid cancer cells, they lack the ability to absorb iodine.

Encapsulated tumor. This refers to a cancerous growth that is completely surrounded by benign cells. Once the tumor has been removed, the pathologist will determine whether it is encapsulated. This type of tumor will influence the follow-up treatments.

Margins. Margins refer to the outer edges of a tumor. When hair-like structures extend outward from the surface, this is called positive margins. When there are no hair-like structures, this is called negative margins. When there is limited growth of these extensions, it is called close margins. During the surgical removal of a tumor, it is difficult for the surgeon to determine the type of margins present since some of these growths may be microscopic in size. Once the tumor has been removed, the pathologist will determine whether it is positive, negative, or close. The type of margin found will influence the follow-up treatments.

Mixture of thyroid cancer cells. Several times pathology reports find different types of cells within a single tumor. The findings may show benign cells with a mix of one or two cancerous types. Treatments for these types of tumors may range widely—from treatments designed to combat the most aggressive thyroid cancer first to prescribing several treatments at once to fight all the cancers.

Tumor size. Tumors are measures in centimeters (cm). A 1 cm is a little smaller than a 1/2-inch; 3 cm is a little bigger than 1 inch; and 5 cm is a little smaller than 2 inches. The size of a tumor may determine the treatment given.

STAGES OF THYROID CANCER

In general, all cancers are classified in terms of how far the cancer has spread. Normally, the location(s), the size of tumors, and the patient's age may determine the stage at, which a cancer has progressed. In some cases, however, the speed at, which a cancer may progress determines its stage. All thyroid cancers have their own specific stages; however, as a general rule of thumb the following factors determine a thyroid cancer's stage.

Stage 0. This refers to an early stage of medullary thyroid cancer in, which a specialized screening test indicates the presents of medullary cells with no physical thyroid tumor being detected.

Stage I. The tumor is found inside of the thyroid with or without limited spread to nearby tissues and lymph nodes.

Stage II. The tumor is found inside the thyroid and has metastasized to other parts of the body. The tumor itself is small, 2 cm in size or smaller.

Stage III. The tumor is found inside the thyroid and has metastasized to other parts of the body. The tumor may be 2 cm to 4 cm in size or greater.

Stage IV. The tumor is found inside the thyroid and is now widespread throughout the body. However, in the case of anaplastic and undifferentiated thyroid cancer, any finding of this type of cancer is immediately classified as stage IV whether or not it has spread.

STANDARD TREATMENTS

The treatment of patients with thyroid cancer is often multidisciplinary involving surgeons, endocrinologists, medical oncologists, and nuclear medicine radiologists. Each type of thyroid cancer has its own treatment steps called protocols. While these protocols may differ in duration, sequence, and/or dosage based upon the individual patients, the following treatments are most common.

Surgery

In a *lobectomy*, only the side containing the tumor is removed. In a *partial thyroidectomy*, the majority of the thyroid is removed leaving only a small section in place. In a *total thyroidectomy* the entire thyroid is taken out. If there is evidence that any of the nearby lymph nodes contain cancer cells, a *lymph node dissection* is performed. In patients with metastatic differentiated thyroid cancer, total thyroidectomy with or without compartment-oriented lymph node dissection is still recommended to facilitate the use of radioiodine therapy and to reduce locoregional morbidity (the cancer comes back in the primary site or nearby lymph nodes) from tumor invasion. The extent of the initial thyroidectomy in patients with low risk, differentiated thyroid cancer (tumor size smaller than 4 cm. without preoperative evidence of invasion in surrounding structures or detectable swollen lymph nodes) remains controversial. The medical literature suggests that a thyroid lobectomy may provide a comparable outcome to a total thyroidectomy if lymph node metastases are detected, compartment-oriented therapeutic lymph node dissection is recommended. Prophylactic central neck lymph node dissection is suggested in individuals with high-risk features for nodal metastasis such as T3-T4 tumors.

Radioactive Iodine (RAI) Ablation

Post-surgical management includes radioactive iodine (RAI) ablation especially for people with high risks for tumor recurrence, patients with metastatic disease, and individuals with persistent or recurrent disease. The benefit of RAI has been demonstrated in patients with a high risk for recurrence. RAI decreases the risk of recurrence and disease-related mortality. However, RAI for low-risk patients is controversial as there is no convincing data demonstrating its effectiveness and clinical benefit. People who have an excellent response after surgery, defined as undetectable thyroglobulin, do not usually require RAI ablation. Radioactive iodine is swallowed in a liquid form or capsule. The RAI is then absorbed into all the functioning thyroid cells. As the RAI is collected within the cells, the concentration of radiation destroys the thyroid gland along with the cancerous cell.

Radiation Therapy

High energy x-rays are focused on a general area of the neck using any number of external radiation machines. In some cases, a small dosage of chemotherapy is given to the patient to enhance the effect of the radiation. This treatment is designed to kill cancer cells and shrink tumors.

Chemotherapy

Chemotherapeutic agents are anti-cancer drugs that may be taken by mouth or injection. These medications are given to kill or shrink tumors. Based on the specific chemo, there may be a number of side effects with some becoming so intense that the chemotherapy must be stopped. Some of the side effects may be short-lived while others may be permanent.

Radiation and Chemotherapy

In some cases, before the radiation session begins, a low dosage of chemotherapy is given to the patient to enhance the effect of the radiation.

In other cases, a full dosage of chemo is given along with the radiation treatments. This type of combination is considered aggressive.

Targeted Drugs

The FDA has approved several drugs specifically designed to combat various thyroid cancers. They work based on disrupting the cancer cells' ability to function. Some do this by cutting off the tumor's blood supply, by interfering with its internal pathways, or by attaching chemicals to its receptors. Some of these drugs are used in conjunction with certain chemotherapies. While still in the early stages, these drugs provide a new weapon against these malignancies.

Clinical Trials

In many medical centers, clinical trials of new and unproven treatments are offered for free to patients who have met certain criteria—perhaps having exhausted all other standard treatments. These clinical trials may include new drugs, new chemotherapies, or a combination of drugs and / or chemotherapeutic agents.

There are four phases of a clinical trial:

- **Phase I** evaluates a treatment for its safety and the best way it can be administered

- **Phase II** determines, which cancer it works best against

- **Phase III** measures its effectiveness compared to similar FDA approved treatments

- **Phase IV** studies the effect of its long–term use as well as its side effects

Before entering any clinical trial, it is wise to ask what phase the trial is in, and what the preliminary results of the trials have shown.

Hormone Therapy

Thyroid hormone replacement after surgical resection is necessary to replace thyroid hormones previously made by the body and to inhibit tumor growth by maintaining low TSH level and thus reducing the risk of recurrence. The clinical benefit of TSH suppression depends on the aggressiveness of the tumor. Recent American Thyroid Association guidelines recommend TSH suppression for patients with high risk (TSH goal:

<0.1 mIU/L) and intermediated risk (TSH goal: 0.1 to 0.5 mIU/L) thyroid cancer. However, thus far no data has demonstrated the benefits of low serum TSH level in patients with low-risk tumors after thyroidectomy.

TYPES OF THYROID CANCERS

Once the type of thyroid cancer has been determined, you may see either an endocrinologist, a doctor specializing in thyroid disorders, and/or an oncologist, a doctor specializing in cancer. With rare and/or aggressive cancers, you would most likely be treated by an oncologist; otherwise, the cancer is usually treated by an endocrinologist. Normally, cancers of the thyroid that are differentiated are very treatable and commonly curable. Tumors that are poorly differentiated are more aggressive and normally require more intensive treatments. The following information will provide a description of the individual types of thyroid cancers as well as their treatments. Some treatments for the same cancers differ based on an individual's age.

PAPILLARY THYROID CANCER (PTC) (PAPILLARY THYROID CARCINOMA)

Papillary thyroid cancer (PTC) cells originate from the uncontrolled growth of follicular cells. Genetically, PTC is driven by activating mutations in *BRAF, RAS*, or *RET/PTC* rearrangements, which activates thyroid cell abnormal proliferation (growth). PTC was the first human cancer to be consistently associated with RET fusions (so called RET/PTC rearrangements). PTC is typically associated with lesions in genes causing unscheduled activation of the MAPK (mitogen-activated protein kinase) cascade. It is referred to as a carcinoma since it begins in the tissue lining the inner or outer surface of the thyroid. This represents approximately 70 to 80 percent of all thyroid cancers, making it the most common form. The vast majority of papillary cancer cells are differentiated.

There are, however, some rare but aggressive variant forms of papillary cancer cells. Aggressive variants of papillary thyroid cancer have been described with increasing frequency. These variants include diffuse sclerosing variant, tall cell variant, columnar cell variant, solid variant, and hobnail variant. They are poorly differentiated. These cells may be mixed in with the differentiated papillary thyroid cancer cells.

Potential Spread

It can spread to the surrounding tissues and lymph nodes. These additional growths in the neck area are called cervical metastasis. Although uncommon, it can spread to the lungs and bones.

Tests

Blood tests, ultrasound, scans, a fine needle aspiration (FNA), and/or a personalized genetic test may be performed.

Treatments

Surgery. Surgery is normally first done to remove the tumor(s). This may require removal of one side of the thyroid gland or the complete thyroid. When surgery cannot be done, radiation therapy is commonly the suggested course of treatment.

Radioactive iodine. After surgery, radioactive iodine (RAI) is given. For RAI therapy to be most effective, you must have a high level of thyroid-stimulating hormone (TSH or thyrotropin) in the blood. This hormone is what makes thyroid tissue (and cancer cells) take up radioactive iodine. If your thyroid has been removed, there are a couple of ways to raise TSH levels before being treated with RAI.

One way is to stop taking thyroid hormone pills for several weeks. This causes very low thyroid hormone levels (hypothyroidism), which makes the pituitary gland release more TSH. This intentional hypothyroidism is temporary, but it often causes symptoms like tiredness, depression, weight gain, constipation, muscle aches, and reduced concentration.

Another way is to get an injection (shot) of thyrotropin (Thyrogen), which can make withholding thyroid hormone for a long period of time unnecessary. This drug is given daily for 2 days, followed by RAI on the third day.

Most doctors also recommend that you follow a low-iodine diet for 1 or 2 weeks before treatment. This means avoiding foods that contain iodized salt and red dye #3, as well as dairy products, eggs, seafood, and soy.

External beam radiation therapy. This therapy may be offered to kill those papillary cancer cells that were not eradicated by the RAI treatment.

Levothyroxine sodium. Once the treatments have been completed, patients will normally be required to take the drug levothyroxine sodium, a synthetic thyroid hormone, for the rest of their lives.

Blood tests. Follow-up blood tests are normally given every 6 to 12 months to check thyroid hormone levels.

Medications. New targeted therapies are available for refractory cancer patients, such as BRAF inhibitors.

OUTCOMES (PROGNOSIS)

The survival rate for this type of cancer is very good with more than 95 percent of adults having a survival rate of at least 10 years. Having check-ups regularly to catch potential reoccurrence is very important since early detection greatly increases survival rates.

FOLLICULAR THYROID CANCER (FOLLICULAR CARCINOMA)

Follicular thyroid cancer represents 10 to 15 percent of all cases of thyroid cancer making it the second most common thyroid cancer after papillary carcinoma but it has more aggressive behavior. A follicular carcinoma develops from the uncontrolled growth of the follicular cell. As with papillary, it is well differentiated. There is also a benign form of this cell called a follicular adenoma, which, in the past, could not be identified when compared to the follicular carcinoma in early tests. The new personalized genetic test may help determine if the follicular cell is malignant.

As with papillary cancer, the follicular cancer cell has its own form of variant cells. That variant form is Hurthle cell thyroid cancer. (See Hurthle Cell Cancer, page 312.)

Potential Spread

Usually, follicular cancer does not spread to the surrounding tissue and lymph nodes. However, while some forms of follicular cancer are minimally invasive, others can be highly aggressive. When aggressive, these cells can spread to all organs throughout the body.

Tests

Early testing using blood tests, ultrasound, scans, and/or a fine needle aspiration (FNA) can identify the growth as coming from the follicular cell. A personalized genetic test may identify the cells as cancerous at an earlier stage; however, standard practice is to remove the tumor through surgery, and have it evaluated by a pathologist, so that the tumor can be accurately identified as follicular thyroid cancer.

Treatments

Surgery. Surgery is normally first done to remove the tumor(s). This may require removal of one side of the thyroid gland or the complete thyroid. Normally, the size of the growth and the patient's age may determine how much of the thyroid gland is removed. When surgery cannot be done, the patient may receive radiation therapy.

Radioactive iodine. After surgery, radioactive iodine (RAI) is given. For RAI therapy to be most effective, you must have a high level of thyroid-stimulating hormone (TSH or thyrotropin) in the blood. This hormone is what makes thyroid tissue (and cancer cells) take up radioactive iodine. If your thyroid has been removed, there are a couple of ways to raise TSH levels before being treated with RAI.

One way is to stop taking thyroid hormone pills for several weeks. This causes very low thyroid hormone levels (hypothyroidism), which makes the pituitary gland release more TSH. This intentional hypothyroidism is temporary, but it often causes symptoms like tiredness, depression, weight gain, constipation, muscle aches, and reduced concentration.

Another way is to get an injection (shot) of thyrotropin (Thyrogen), which can make withholding thyroid hormone for a long period of time unnecessary. This drug is given daily for 2 days, followed by RAI on the third day.

Most doctors also recommend that you follow a low-iodine diet for 1 or 2 weeks before treatment. This means avoiding foods that contain iodized salt and red dye #3, as well as dairy products, eggs, seafood, and soy.

External beam radiation therapy. Based on the extent of the tumor and the effect of RAI treatment on the follicular cancer cells, external beam radiation therapy may be offered to kill the remaining cancer cells.

Levothyroxine sodium. Once the treatment has been completed, patients will normally be required to take the drug levothyroxine sodium, a synthetic thyroid hormone, for the rest of their lives.

Blood tests. Follow-up blood tests are normally given every 6 to 12 months to check on thyroid hormone levels.

Medications. New targeted therapies are available for refractory cancer patients, such as BRAF inhibitors.

OUTCOMES (PROGNOSIS)

The survival rate for this type of cancer is 90 percent when the follicular cells are differentiated, however, the recurrence rate can be as high as 30 percent. Having check-ups regularly to catch potential reoccurrence is very important since early detection greatly increases survival rates.

HURTHLE CELL THYROID CANCER (HURTHLE CELL CARCINOMA)

Because Hurthle cell thyroid cancer is a variant form of follicular thyroid cell, it is classified under follicular thyroid cancer. Hurthle cell is considered a rare cancer, accounting for 5 to 10 percent of differentiated thyroid cancers. When a follicular cell turns into a Hurthle cell, it takes on a vastly different appearance. Unlike normal follicular cells, however, they do not provide a useful service to the body. Hurthle cells may be benign or malignant. Like the follicular growths, the benign form of this cell, called a Hurthle cell adenoma, has been hard to identify when compared to the Hurthle cell carcinoma in early tests. The new personalized genetic test may help determine if the follicular cell is malignant.

An individual having Hashimoto's thyroiditis or Hashimoto's disease may increase the odds of developing Hurthle cells in the thyroid.

Potential Spread

Like follicular cancer, Hurthle cells do not usually spread to the surrounding tissue and lymph nodes. Some Hurthle cells can be minimally invasive, while others can be highly aggressive. When aggressive, these cells can spread to any and all organs throughout the body. While benign Hurthle cell tumors may not be dangerous, and do not usually grow back once removed, some of these benign cells may turn cancerous in rare instances.

Tests

Blood tests, ultrasound, scans, and/or a fine needle aspiration (FNA) can identify the growth as being Hurthle cell. A personalized genetic test may identify the cells as cancerous at an earlier stage; however, standard practice is to remove the tumor through surgery, have it evaluated by a pathologist, so that the tumor can be accurately identified as Hurthle cell.

Treatments

Surgery. Surgery is normally first done to remove the tumor(s). This may require removal of one side of the thyroid gland or the complete thyroid. Normally, the size of the growth and the patient's age may determine how much of the thyroid gland is removed. When surgery cannot be done, the patient may receive radiation therapy.

Radioactive iodine (RAI). After surgery, radioactive iodine (RAI) is given. For RAI therapy to be most effective, you must have a high level of thyroid-stimulating hormone (TSH or thyrotropin) in the blood. This hormone is what makes thyroid tissue (and cancer cells) take up radioactive iodine. If your thyroid has been removed, there are a couple of ways to raise TSH levels before being treated with RAI.

One way is to stop taking thyroid hormone pills for several weeks. This causes very low thyroid hormone levels (hypothyroidism), which makes the pituitary gland release more TSH. This intentional hypothyroidism is temporary, but it often causes symptoms like tiredness, depression, weight gain, constipation, muscle aches, and reduced concentration.

Another way is to get an injection (shot) of thyrotropin (Thyrogen), which can make withholding thyroid hormone for a long period of time unnecessary. This drug is given daily for 2 days, followed by RAI on the third day.

Most doctors also recommend that you follow a low-iodine diet for 1 or 2 weeks before treatment. This means avoiding foods that contain iodized salt and red dye #3, as well as dairy products, eggs, seafood, and soy.

External beam radiation therapy. Based on the extent of the tumor and the effect of RAI treatment on the Hurthle cells, external beam radiation therapy may be offered to kill the remaining cancer cells.

Levothyroxine sodium. Once the treatment has been completed, patients will normally be required to take the drug levothyroxine sodium, a synthetic thyroid hormone, for the rest of their lives.

Blood tests. Follow-up blood tests are normally given every 6 to 12 months to check on thyroid hormone levels.

Medications. New targeted therapies are available for refractory cancer patients, such as BRAF inhibitors.

OUTCOMES (PROGNOSIS)

Statistics indicate that the survival rate for this type of cancer may be correlated to the age of the patient, the size of the tumor, how differentiated the cells are, and whether or not the tumor has metastasized. Usually, the younger the patient and smaller the tumor, the better the outcome. Older patients with metastasis may be at a disadvantage, however, in rare cancers such as this, survival rates are best evaluated on a case-by-case basis.

MEDULLARY THYROID CANCER (MEDULLARY CARCINOMA)

Medullary thyroid cancer (MTC) originates from the parafollicular cells (also called C cells) of the thyroid. Though statistically low in numbers, they are the third most common thyroid cancer making up 3 to 10 percent of all thyroid cancers. This type of cancer cell is less differentiated than papillary and follicular.

Normal parafollicular cells secrete a number of hormones, including calcitonin, ACTH, serotonin, prostaglandins, and vasoactive intestinal peptide (VIP). When the parafollicular cells change into medullary cancer cells, however, they produce larger and larger amounts of these hormones as they increase in numbers. This may create several health issues, including high levels of calcitonin and diarrhea.

There are two types of medullary thyroid cancers. One is *sporadic MTC*, which does not run in families, and the second is *inherited MTC*. Sporadic MTC accounts for 75 to 80 percent of all medullary thyroid cancers. Inherited MTC, which accounts for the remaining 20 to 25 percent, may include a group of other endocrine disorders.

These disorders may become evident in a variety of symptoms associated with each affected endocrine gland. Inherited mutations in a gene called RET (rearranged during transfection—when DNA or RNA is artificially inserted into the gene) have been associated with the development of medullary thyroid cancers, and account for approximately one out of four cases. This condition is known as familial medullary thyroid cancer (FMTC). Since the discovery of the RET receptor tyrosine kinase in 1985, alterations of this protein have been found in diverse thyroid cancer subtypes. RET gene rearrangements are observed in papillary thyroid carcinoma, which result in RET fusion products. By contrast, single amino acid substitutions and small insertions and/or deletions are typical of hereditary and sporadic medullary thyroid carcinoma.

Potential Spread

Initially, medullary tumors tend to be located in the back of the thyroid gland, closer to the larynx and trachea. Therefore, as it grows it may commonly compress or invade the throat area resulting in hoarseness or respiratory difficulty. It may also spread to nearby lymph nodes. While there may be a lower percentage of metastasis spreading to other parts of the body, when it does occur, the common areas include the chest cavity, liver, lungs, and bones.

Tests

Blood tests, ultrasound, scans, a fine needle aspiration (FNA), and/or personalized genetic test may be performed.

Treatments

Surgery. Surgery is normally first done to remove the tumor(s). This may require removal of one side of the thyroid gland, or the complete thyroid based upon the tumor's involvement with the structures around it.

Radioactive iodine (RAI). After surgery, radioactive iodine (RAI) is usually *not* given. Because the medullary cell does not readily absorb iodine, RAI has little effect on this type of thyroid cancer.

External beam radiation therapy. External beam radiation may be utilized, however the use of it must be based on the individual case.

Chemotherapy. Standard chemotherapy may be an option; however, such treatments have shown limited effectiveness.

Medications. There are new targeted drugs available that are aimed at blocking the pathways necessary to the development and progression of medullary cancer cells. Two small-molecule tyrosine kinase inhibitors, Vandetanib and Cabozantinib, are currently available as approved agents for the treatment of advanced or progressive MTC and provide significant increases in progression-free survival. You can learn more about these drugs from your oncologist and also at the end of this chapter.

Levothyroxine sodium. Once the treatment has been completed, patients will normally be required to take the drug levothyroxine sodium, a synthetic thyroid hormone, for the rest of their lives.

Blood tests. Follow-up blood tests are normally given every 6 to 12 months to check on thyroid hormone levels.

OUTCOMES (PROGNOSIS)

Patients with disease limited to only the thyroid gland, without nodal involvement, have a very low risk for recurrence and rarely die from their disease. However, individuals with nodal involvement are at a higher risk for recurrence or persistent disease. Overall, the outcome for patients with MTC is good. The 10-year survival rate for MTC patients is 75 to 85 percent.

ANAPLASTIC THYROID CANCER (ATC) AND POORLY DIFFERENTIATED THYROID CANCER (PDTC)

Anaplastic thyroid cancer (ATC) is a rare and aggressive cancer. It occurs in approximately 1 to 2 percent of thyroid cancer patients. While it is thought to be a variant form of papillary thyroid cancer, because it is undifferentiated, it is difficult to tell its origin. Since it is a rapidly growing cancer, once it has been determined that the cells are ATC, it needs to be treated quickly. Based on its aggressive behavior, ATC is classified as being Stage IV upon identification. Initially, ATC is harder to detect since it can grow unnoticed until a lump in the neck is observed or some hoarseness in the voice is heard. It may also be present with other types of thyroid cancers.

There is another cancer cell called poorly differentiated thyroid carcinoma (PDTC), which looks like and behaves in a similar manner as anaplastic thyroid cancer. It too is aggressive and, as its name indicates, poorly differentiated. While it is difficult to identify PDTC from ATC in its early stages, as the tumor grows they differ from each other in appearance and smell according to surgeons who have operated on these two forms of cancer. PDTC and ATC are normally treated in the same manner.

Potential Spread

Anaplastic thyroid cancer is likely to spread to nearby lymph nodes. As it increases in size, it grows towards the larynx, trachea, and esophagus. It may commonly compress or invade the throat area resulting in hoarseness or respiratory difficulty. When it is discovered later in its development, it commonly spreads to the lungs and/or bones.

Tests

Ultrasound, scans, and/or a fine needle aspiration (FNA) may be performed. Because ATC is so rare, the initial FNA pathology results may be described as poorly differentiated cells, however, if it is not identified as ATC or of a cancerous nature, more tests should be done immediately.

Treatments

Because anaplastic thyroid cancer occurs so rarely, it is important to find a medical center that has had experience dealing with this form of cancer. (See Resources on page 329.)

Surgery. Surgery is normally first done to remove the tumor(s). This may require removal of one side of the thyroid gland, or the complete thyroid based upon the tumor's involvement with the structures around it. Based upon how extensive the growth of the ATC is around the trachea, and esophagus, a tracheotomy may be performed to allow for easier breathing and a feeding tube inserted.

When there is extensive tumor growth around the structures in the neck, surgery may not be an option. In such cases, chemotherapy and/or external beam radiation may be used to shrink the tumor.

Radioactive iodine (RAI). Radioactive iodine (RAI) is *not* an option. Because ATC cells do not absorb iodine, RAI has little effect on this type of thyroid cancer.

External beam radiation therapy. After surgery, external beam radiation treatments are normally given. In some cases, a low dose of chemotherapy is included to enhance the effects of the radiation. The drug docetaxel, when used in conjunction with radiation, has shown some effectiveness. Based on the length of this treatment, having a feeding tube inserted may be suggested.

Chemotherapy. A combination of chemotherapeutic agents may be an option; however, such treatments have shown very limited effectiveness with one exception. ATC patients with the BRAF gene mutation showed positive results when given the combination of vemurafenib and dabrafenib.

Medications. While there are several new targeted drugs available that are aimed at blocking the pathways necessary to the development and progression of the ATC cells, their effectiveness is limited. You can learn more about these drugs from your oncologist. Also see the end of this chapter for further discussion.

Clinical trials. There are a few clinical trials available for ATC patients. (See Resources on page 329 for more information.) Before entering any clinical trial, however, it is wise to ask what phase the trial is in, and what the preliminary results of the trials have shown.

Levothyroxine sodium. Once treatments have been completed, patients will normally be required to take the drug levothyroxine sodium, a synthetic thyroid hormone, for the rest of their lives.

Blood tests. Follow-up blood tests are normally given every 6 to 12 months to check on thyroid hormone levels.

OUTCOMES (PROGNOSIS)

Patients who are able to identify this type of cancer early in its progression, with tumors that have little involvement around the structures in the neck, have a higher rate of survival. Unfortunately, in many cases, ATC becomes notable only after it has progressed to an advanced stage. Because of this, it is a difficult cancer to treat successfully.

NEW THERAPIES FOR ADVANCED THYROID CANCER

The significant scientific advances in the molecular characterization of thyroid cancer raised the use of more targeted therapies for advanced cancers, such as tyrosine kinase inhibitors and anti-angiogenic drugs. Recently, several novel drugs that target cell proliferation, angiogenesis, apoptosis, immunosuppression, metabolomic reprogramming, and epigenetic changes have been tested.

In addition to targeted therapies, immunotherapy by targeting PD-/PDL-1 axis (a protein that keeps the body's immune responses under control) showed a reduction of tumor growth in several pre-clinical models of aggressive thyroid cancer.

Targeted Therapies Against MAPK Pathway

Mitogen-Activated Protein Kinase (MAPK) pathways connect extracellular signals to the network that controls cell proliferation, motility, and cell death. Thyroid cancer often presents genetic alterations that activate the MAPK pathway. Vemurafenib and dabrafenib are BRAF^{V600E} inhibitors that function as ATP-competitive inhibitors. Selumetinib is a potent non-ATP competitive MEK1/2 inhibitor.

Targeting of PI3K/Akt Pathway

The PI3K/Akt pathway plays a crucial role in thyroid carcinogenesis, cell dedifferentiation, invasion, and metastasis. The three main players of these pathways are PI3K, Akt, and mTOR. Everolimus is a kinase inhibitor used in RAI-refractory thyroid cancer. It targets mTOR.

Anti-Angiogenic TKI

Sorafenib is a multikinase inhibitor that targets VEGFR 1,2 and 3, RET, FLT3, c-Kit, BRAF, and BRAF^{V600E}. It is approved for patients with advanced, iodine-refractory thyroid cancer. Lenvatinib is a multikinase inhibitor, targeting VEGFR1-3, FGFR, PDGFR, RET, and KIT

Immunotherapy

The interactions between the tumor microenvironment and cancer cells are involved in cancer progression. The increasing findings regarding the mechanisms underlying the ability of cancer cells to escape the immune response surveillance have made the immune system a new promising therapeutic target in oncology. Analysis of the Immunoscore, a method to estimate the prognosis of patients with cancer based on the infiltrative immune cells in cancer, of 505 patients with thyroid cancer, revealed a significant negative correlation between thyroid differentiation score and immunosuppressive markers such as CTLA-4 and PD-L1. The anti-PD-1 antibody Pembrolizumab is now currently being used to treat refractory thyroid cancer.

In addition, a combination of PLX4720, a $BRAF^{V600E}$ inhibitor and anti-PD-L1/PD-1 antibody in a preclinical model of ATC, reduced the tumor growth, and increased in tumor CD8+ cytotoxic T cells, FoxP3+ Tregs, and natural killer (NK) cells, thus demonstrating an induction of the immunosuppressive tumor microenvironment. Taken together, these findings suggest that a combination therapy of $BRAF^{V600E}$ inhibitor and anti- PD-1/PD-L1 antibody is a promising therapeutic strategy for metastatic thyroid cancer.

RET-Positive Thyroid Cancer New Therapies

As you have seen, advanced thyroid cancer can be driven by a gene in your body. One of those genes is RET. Retevmo is available for RET-positive advanced thyroid cancer. Retevmo was studied in the largest clinical trial of people with RET-positive cancers. The trial included 373 people with advanced thyroid cancer (including medullary, papillary, poorly differentiated, anaplastic, and Hurthle cell), and 170 had tumors that were eligible to be evaluated for shrinkage. The trial evaluated how many people responded to treatment, which means their tumors either shrank or disappeared completely and how long the response lasted. Retevmo has been shown to shrink tumors in the majority of people with other RET-positive advanced thyroid cancers. It is also known as Selpercatinib. Retevmo may affect both healthy cells and tumor cells, which can result in side effects, some of, which can be serious.

RETEVMO may cause serious side effects, including heart rhythm changes, liver problems, lung problems, high blood pressure, abnormal bleeding, allergic reactions, tumor lysis syndrome (which can cause you to have kidney failure), poor wound healing, hypothyroidism, decreased white blood count, decreased levels of sodium in the blood, decreased levels of calcium in the blood, and may cause infertility. The most common side effects of RETEVMO include:

- Abdominal (stomach) pain
- Constipation
- Diarrhea
- Dry mouth
- Fatigue
- Headache

- Hypertension (high blood pressure)
- Nausea
- Rash
- Swelling of your arms, legs, hands, and feet (edema)

OTHER CANCERS OF THE THYROID

The thyroid gland may also be the site of other types of cancers, such as the lung, kidney, and breast that have spread (metastasized) from other parts of the body. On the other hand, the thyroid may rarely be the site of metastasis from other primary tumors, which include sarcomas, lymphomas, epidermoid carcinomas, and teratomas—a type of germ cell tumor that may contain several different kinds of tissue, such as hair, muscle, and bone.

Tests

Blood tests, ultrasound, scans, a fine needle aspiration (FNA), and/or personalized genetic test may be performed to determine the type of cancer it is.

Treatments

Once the specific type of cancer has been determined, work with your endocrinologist and oncologist specializing in that type of cancer.

Suggestions

The stark reality is that over 60,000 people will be told that they have thyroid cancer this year—and sitting there, in a doctor's office, being told you have any type of cancer is not easy. The news tends to knock the wind right out of you. While the vast majority of thyroid cancer patients will be treated successfully, there are important things that a patient should consider doing in preparation for the journey that lies ahead of them. These same suggestions also hold true for those patients with more aggressive thyroid cancers. The better prepared you are, the better decisions you will be able to make.

Find the Right Advocate

An advocate is someone who will not only be with you as you go through the various stages of the process, but also ask questions and take notes when necessary. Most people, upon being told they have cancer, may hear the doctor talking, but they are in shock, and unable to respond appropriately, or remember what is being said. Therefore, choosing the right advocate is important. Whether it's an adult child, spouse, parent, or friend, make sure that they have the time to be there with you, and that they will not be overwhelmed by the process.

If you don't have anyone that you can rely on, reach out to cancer support groups. They can be found online. They may be part of a

Hyperthyroidism and Cancer

Certain types of cancer cells can create an overproduction of thyroid hormones, which can lead to hyperthyroidism, along with all of its signs and symptoms. (See page 75.) This can occur due to a pituitary tumor producing too much TSH or to thyroid cancer cells, capable of producing hormones, overproducing thyroid hormones. While these conditions are uncommon, it is important to be aware of them. They include:

TSH-secreting Pituitary Adenomas

These are rare, slow growing pituitary tumors and account for about 1 to 2 percent of all pituitary adenomas that are removed through surgery. These tumors can be aggressive and invasive. They may also be a cause of hyperthyroidism.

Struma Ovarii

Struma ovarii is a rare tumor that occurs in a teratoma or dermoid of the ovary. It comprises about 1 percent of all ovarian tumors. It is often mixed with a carcinoid tumor and can occur in association with multiple endocrine neoplasia type IIA. The cause of struma ovarii is not known. Eight percent are benign, and 90 percent are localized. Treatment is removal of the ovarian tumor. If the individual is thyrotoxic before surgery, then thionamides are given. B-adrenergic blocking medications may also need to be prescribed.

nonprofit cancer group, or they may be affiliated with a medical center. (See Resources on page 329.) Many groups have volunteers that can be of assistance.

Learn as Much as You Can and Ask Questions

Making informed decisions is not always easy. The easiest path for some is to simply follow the instructions given by your doctor. Certainly, it is important to what your doctor has to offer, however, you and/or your advocate should learn as much about the disease and your treatment options as possible. Too many people are afraid to ask questions.

There are various hard questions to ask such as: What are my chances of survival if I do this or do that? Are there any side effects from the treatments? Is there anything I can do to improve my odds? Have you treated this type of cancer before? When you don't understand, something being

Thyrotoxicosis Caused By Pregnancy and Trophoblastic Disease

Human chorionic gonadotropin (HCG) is a hormone that is produced in a pregnant woman. It has intrinsic TSH-like activity. In about 2 to 3 percent of normal pregnancies, gestational transient thyrotoxicosis is present due to elevated HCG concentrations. Familial gestational hyperthyroidism can also occur due to a gene mutation, which makes the body hypersensitive to HCG. Thyrotoxicosis can also be induced by molar pregnancy and by trophoblastic disease in both men and women. In a molar pregnancy with hyperthyroidism, studies have shown that when the hydatidiform mole is removed, the thyrotoxicosis resolves.

Thyrotoxicosis Caused By Metastatic Differentiated Thyroid Carcinoma

Thyrotoxicosis caused by functioning metastasis of differentiated thyroid carcinoma is uncommon. Eighty-five percent of the people are over the age of 40, and it is more common in women than men. The clinical picture is the same for this disease as it is for other causes of thyrotoxicosis. Excessive thyroid hormone production is due to the large mass of metastatic tissue. Treatment is surgery or radioactive iodine.

told to you, tell them you don't understand, and ask them to explain it to you in simpler language. If you feel you are not satisfied with the information you are getting, do not hesitate to get second or third opinions from other healthcare professionals.

Be Prepared

It has been the Boy Scouts' motto for over one hundred years and there's a good reason why it should be yours. You need to be prepared for what lies in ahead of you. There are a number of important things to consider:

- Always take copies of all your test results with you on your visits to doctors or medical centers, especially if you are visiting them for the first time. If a past scan is available only in an electronic form, have the laboratory provide you with a copy on a CD. You will find that it is a standard practice for doctors to request laboratory reports be sent to them before your visit. However, many times you show up, but the reports have not. Be prepared!

- Learn as much as you can about any procedures that you will be undergoing. Whether it's a scan, an insertion of a feeding tube, an operation, the necessary preparation for radiation—learn what's involved. For example, some scans involve being put into a tubular enclosure. If this is a problem for you, ask if they have an open scanner, or perhaps ask for something to calm you down. Also, ask how long these procedures take. It's helpful to know since you now must work your life around their schedules. Be prepared!

- Ask questions about any and all of the possible side effects of any procedure. Over the years, many drugs have been developed to either overcome or lessen side effects. There may also be natural remedies that might help alleviate some of these problems. Know what remedies are out there ahead of time. Be prepared!

- Take things to do with you while you wait. Read a book, take an iPad, listen to music, do a crossword puzzle, text a friend—take something along that can help pass the time. As you will discover, there is a reason they are called waiting rooms, so be prepared!

- Consider joining a thyroid cancer listserv. The term listserv refers to online groups devoted to working with thyroid cancer patients and their advocates. These groups are normally composed of current patients, survivors, advocates, and in some cases, medical professionals who can answer your questions about almost anything related to your situation. They can provide information based upon their own experiences. They can likewise be a source of great support in understanding that you are not alone. (See Resources on page 329.) Be prepared!

It is not uncommon for you to feel as though you are not in control of your present circumstances. The suggestions above should help to empower you as a patient. By preparing in advance—by knowing what to ask and what to do—you will find that you do have some control over the process.

CONCLUSION

I have heard it said that if you are going to get cancer, thyroid cancer is the best one to get. Personally, I don't think any cancer fits that description. What I will say is that modern medicine has been able to treat the vast majority of thyroid cancers successfully. Additionally, some of the new genetic tests allow patients to learn relatively quickly whether a node is benign or malignant. However, there are enough rare and aggressive forms of these cancers to make the journey that much more difficult. The great news is that there are new medications that have been shown to be very effective for the more aggressive forms of thyroid cancer.

Interestingly, most of thyroid diseases show female predilection, especially autoimmune thyroid diseases and thyroid cancer. Recently, the local expression of ER (estrogen receptors) subtypes and their individual mediated actions in the pathogenesis of thyroid cancer have received much attention. ER-alpha activation seems to exacerbate the development of thyroid cancer, while wild-type ER-beta plays a protective role against thyroid cancer. Furthermore, estrogen is involved in the regulation of angiogenesis and metastasis that are critical for the outcome of thyroid cancer. In contrast to other carcinomas, however, detailed knowledge on this regulation is still missing for thyroid cancer. Estrogen's relationship to thyroid cancer is an area of current study in the medical literature.

If there is one key to beating thyroid cancer, it is to find it early, take immediate action, and to consider the spiritual component of your life. Therefore, make sure your tests and treatments don't rely on someone else's timetable. I hope the information in this chapter equips you with the appropriate questions in making the decisions that are right for you.

Conclusion

Hopefully by now, you have come to understand the critical role that the thyroid gland and its hormones play in your ability to think, to feel, and to sustain the many systems that keep you alive and functioning normally. As you have seen in the chapters of this book, when the thyroid gland does not function correctly, it can cause any number of serious problems. Too often, the underlying cause of these difficulties goes undetected.

The purpose of my writing this book has been to provide you with a clear understanding of how the thyroid gland works and what thyroid hormones do to keep the body functioning optimally. Literally tens of thousands of men and women suffer from a wide variety of thyroid related health issues and are unaware of the source of their symptoms and signs. Because their condition may be subclinical—in other words, it may not be detected by physical examinations or standard blood tests—patients are sometimes prescribed drugs that are not thyroid hormones to diminish their overt symptoms. Add to that the fact that the number of people with thyroid problems is rapidly growing, and you can see the difficulty that lies ahead for so many individuals.

If you or a loved one suffers from some of the symptoms described in this book, and you have not been able to isolate their cause, I hope you consider acting as an advocate and asking your healthcare provider to determine if these ailments are thyroid related. If, on the other hand, you have been diagnosed with a thyroid issue that is covered in this book, I hope I have been able to provide you with a clearer understanding of what the problem is and how it can be treated. Knowledge is power, and your ability to ask the right questions and understand the answers will, in turn, enable you to make informed decisions about your health.

Always be aware that medicine is a rapidly changing science, and that while I have done my best to provide you with up-to-date information, new tests, and treatments are always emerging. View this book as a springboard to further investigation and be certain that you have all the available facts before making a decision regarding treatment. As long as you understand that you have a significant role to play in overcoming your thyroid disorder, you will have taken an important step toward optimal health.

Resources

American Academy of Anti-Aging Medicine (A4M)
561-997-0112
www.a4m.com
info@a4m.com

The Academy of Anti-Aging Medicine (A4M) is the established global leader for continuing medical education in longevity medicine, metabolic resilience, and whole-person care.

CANCER ORGANIZATIONS

American Thyroid Association
6066 Leesburg Pike, Suite 550 Falls Church, Virginia 22041
703-998-8890
www.thyroid.org
thyroid@thyroid.org
The American Thyroid Association is devoted to thyroid biology and the prevention and treatment of thyroid disease through research, clinical care, education, and public health.

National Cancer Institute (NCI)
800-422-6237
www.cancer.gov
NCIinfo@nih.gov
The National Cancer Institute provides information on all types of cancers, including thyroid cancer. In addition to explaining what these cancers are and how they are normally treated, it offers a listing of clinical trials taking place throughout the country.

ThyCa: Thyroid Cancer Survivors' Association, Inc.
PO Box 1102
Olney, MD 20830-1102
877-588-7904
www.thyca.org
thyca@thyca.org
This nonprofit organization provides information to educate patients and their families about all types and aspects of thyroid cancer, including clinical trial information, medical specialists, and the contacts for other thyroid cancer-related organizations.

City of Hope
1500 East Duarte Road
Duarte, CA 91010
888-641-4652
www.cityofhope.org

*City of Hope is dedicated to making
a difference in the lives of people
with cancer, diabetes, and other life-
threatening illnesses.*

COMPOUNDING PHARMACIES

Compounding is the practice of creating personalized medications to fill in
the gaps left by mass-produced medicine. To meet the special needs of an
individual, a compounding pharmacy can provide unique dosages, innovative delivery methods, and unusual flavorings, and can also eliminate
allergens and unnecessary fillers.

**Professional Compounding
Centers of America (PCCA)**
9901 South Wilcrest Drive Houston,
TX 77099
800-331-2498
www.pccarx.com
*The PCCA supports the creation of
personalized medicine and innovative
products that make a difference in
patients' lives.*

**Alliance for Pharmacy
Compounding (APC)**
100 Daingerfield Rd, Ste 100
Alexandria, VA 22314
281-933-8400
www.a4pc.org
info@a4pc.org
*The Alliance for Pharmacy Compounding
is the voice for pharmacy compounding,
representing compounding pharmacists
and technicians in both 503A and 503B
settings, as well as prescribers, educators,
patients, and suppliers.*

DIAGNOSTIC LABORATORIES

Medical testing now makes it possible to measure your amino acids, fatty
acids, organic acids, vitamin levels, hormone levels, gastrointestinal function, genome, and much more. This means that your regimen can be personalized to meet your specific needs. The following laboratories can perform
tests to evaluate many important aspects of your health. Before ordering any
medical test, be sure to consult with your healthcare practitioner.

Access Medical Labs
5151 Corporate Way
Jupiter, FL 33458

866-720-8386 x120
www.accessmedlab.com

Cyrex Laboratories
2602 South 24th Street
Phoenix, AZ 85034
877-772-9739 (US)
844-216-4763 (Canada)
www.cyrexlabs.com

Doctor's Data
3755 Illinois Avenue
St. Charles, IL 60174
800-323-2784
www.doctorsdata.com

Genova Diagnostics
63 Zillicoa Street
Asheville, NC 28801
800-522-4762
www.gdx.net

Great Plains Laboratory
11813 West 77th Street
Lenexa, KS 66214
800-288-3383
www.greatplainslaboratory.com

Lake Nona Diagnostics
6555 Sanger Rd., Suite 233
Orlando, FL 32827
754-227-7006
www.lakenonadx.com

Microbiome Labs Research Center
1332 Waukegan Rd.
Glenview, IL 60025
904-940-2208
www.biomeFx.com

Rocky Mountain Analytical
105–32 Royal Vista Drive NW
Calgary, Alberta T3R 0H9 Canada
866-370-5227
www.rmalab.com

Rupa Health
www.rupahealth.com

ZRT Laboratory
8605 SW Creekside Place
Beaverton, OR 97008
866-600-1636
www.zrtlab.com

PHARMACEUTICAL-GRADE SUPPLEMENTS

You can find many good supplement brands at health food stores. Always make sure you buy pharmaceutical grade nutrients. The following pharmaceutical grade companies offer many quality nutritional supplements. Contact them for full product lists as well as for directions on ordering their products.

Biotics Research Corporation
6801 Biotics Research Drive
Rosenberg, TX 77471
800-231-5777
www.bioticsresearch.com

Designs for Health, Inc.
980 South Street
Suffield, CT 06078

800-847–8302
www.designsforhealth.com

Douglas Laboratories
112 Technology Drive
Pittsburgh, PA 15275
800-245–4440
www.douglaslabs.com

Metagenics
25 Enterprise
Aliso Viejo, CA 92656
800-692-9400
www.metagenics.com

Microbiome Labs
1332 Waukegan Rd.
Glenview, IL 60025
904-940-2208
https://microbiomelabs.com

Ortho Molecular Products
1991 Duncan Place
Woodstock, IL 60098
800-332–2351
www.orthomolecularproducts.com

Researched Nutritionals
PO Box 224
Los Olivos, CA 93441
800-755-3402
www.researchnutritionals.com

Vital Nutrients
45 Kenneth Dooley Drive
Middletown, CT 06457
888-328–9992
www.vitalnutrients.net

Xymogen
6900 Kingspointe Parkway
Orlando, FL 32819
800-647–6100
www.xymogen.com

References

The information and recommendations presented in this book are based on over a thousand scientific studies, academic papers, and books. If the references for all these sources were printed here, they would add considerable bulk to the book and make it more expensive, as well. For this reason, the publisher and I have decided to present a complete list of references, categorized by section and topic, on the publisher's website. This format has the added advantage of enabling us to make you aware of further important studies and papers as they become available. You can find the references under the listing of my book at www.squareone-publishers.com.

About the Author

Pamela Wartian Smith, MD, MPH, MS, spent her first twenty years of practice as an emergency room physician with the Detroit Medical Center in a level 1 trauma center, and then twenty-eight years as an Anti-Aging/Personalized Medicine specialist. She holds a master's degree in Public Health along with a master's degree in Metabolic and Nutritional Medicine, and is a diplomat of the Board of the American Academy of Anti-Aging Physicians.

Dr. Smith is the founder of the Fellowship in Anti-Aging, Regenerative, and Functional Medicine; co-director of Personalized Medicine Certification at the University of South Florida Morsani College of Medicine; and senior partner for the Center for Personalized Medicine, with offices in Michigan and Florida.

An internationally known speaker on the subject of Anti-Aging/Personalized Medicine, Dr. Smith has been featured on television programs such as the PBS series *The Embrace of Aging* and in numerous magazines, and has hosted two radio shows. She is also the author of fourteen best-selling books, including *What You Must Know About Vitamins, Minerals, Herbs, and So Much More; Max Your Immunity; What You Must Know About Women's Hormones;* and *Maximize Your Male Hormones.*

Index

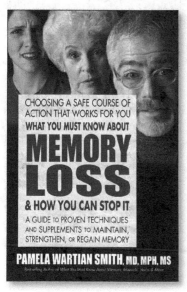
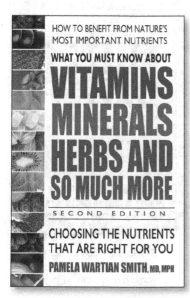
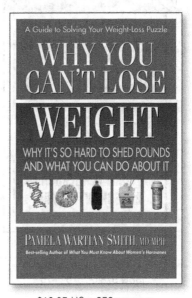

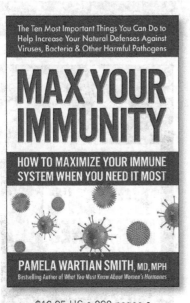
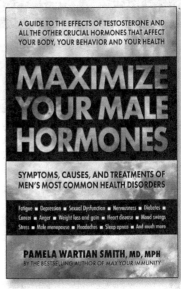
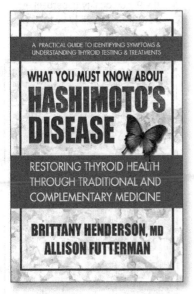
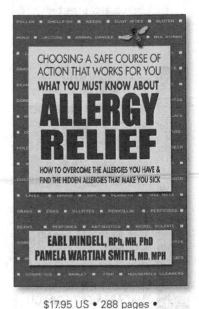